Treating Addiction to Tobacco and Nicotine Products

Treating Addiction to Tobacco and Nicotine Products

by

Jill M. Williams, M.D.
Jonathan Foulds, Ph.D.

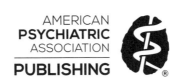

AMERICAN
PSYCHIATRIC
ASSOCIATION
PUBLISHING

If you wish to buy 50 or more copies of the same title, please go to www.appi .org/specialdiscounts for more information.

Copyright © 2025 American Psychiatric Association Publishing
ALL RIGHTS RESERVED

First Edition

Manufactured in the United States of America on acid-free paper

28   27   26   25   24   5   4   3   2   1

American Psychiatric Association Publishing
800 Maine Avenue SW, Suite 900
Washington, DC 20024–2812

www.appi.org

Library of Congress Cataloging-in-Publication Data

Names: Williams, Jill M. (Jill Marie), author. | Foulds, Jonathan, author.
Title: Treating addiction to tobacco and nicotine products / by Jill M. Williams, Jonathan Foulds.
Description: First edition. | Washington, D.C. : American Psychiatric Association Publishing, [2025] | Includes bibliographical references and index.
Identifiers: LCCN 2024029131 (print) | LCCN 2024029132 (ebook) | ISBN 9781615374687 (paperback ; alk. paper) | ISBN 9781615374694 (ebook)
Subjects: MESH: Tobacco Use Disorder–therapy | Tobacco Products–adverse effects | Tobacco Use Disorder–epidemiology | United States–epidemiology
Classification: LCC RA1242.T6 (print) | LCC RA1242.T6 (ebook) | NLM WM 290 | DDC 362.29/6–dc23/eng/20240801
LC record available at https://lccn.loc.gov/2024029131
LC ebook record available at https://lccn.loc.gov/2024029132

British Library Cataloguing in Publication Data

A CIP record is available from the British Library.

Contents

About the Authors

The authors have extensive experience in treating tobacco use disorder as well as in training health care professionals how to intervene using evidence-based practices.

Jill M. Williams, M.D., is a Professor of Psychiatry and Director of the Division of Addiction Psychiatry at the Rutgers University–Robert Wood Johnson Medical School in New Brunswick, New Jersey. She is a past Chair of the APA Council on Addiction Psychiatry. The focus of Dr. Williams' work has been on addressing tobacco use in individuals with mental illness or other addictions through treatment and systems interventions. She is an accomplished academic researcher with more than 100 peer-reviewed publications on tobacco use and behavioral health to her credit. Her approach has been broadly based and translational, ranging from studies of smoking behavior, clinical trials, educational curricula, systems change interventions, epidemiological studies, and policy-based approaches. Dr. Williams has also developed modified training programs for psychiatrists and mental health professionals that result in the increased delivery of tobacco treatment services. She serves as Medical Director for the CHOICES (njchoices.org) and TCTTAC (https://nyctcttac.org) programs.

Jonathan Foulds, Ph.D., is a Professor of Public Health Sciences and Psychiatry at Penn State University College of Medicine. He trained as a clinical psychologist at the University of Glasgow and obtained his Ph.D. at the Institute of Psychiatry at the University of London. He has spent most of his career developing and evaluating methods to help people who smoke beat their addiction to tobacco. He was a founding member and vice president of the Association for the Treatment of Tobacco Use and Dependence (ATTUD). He has been a principal investigator on grants totaling more than $50 million, has published more than 200 scientific papers and book chapters on tobacco and nicotine, and has been invited to speak on smoking cessation in more than

17 countries. He is co-director of the Penn State Center for Research on Tobacco and Health in Hershey, Pennsylvania, where he teaches on smoking cessation and conducts research on tobacco and health.

Disclosures

American Psychiatric Association requires authors to disclose potential conflicts of interest during the time frame (typically about a year) in which they worked on the book. However, the authors have selected to provide more detailed conflict statements.

Jill M. Williams has not done any paid work for tobacco or electronic cigarette manufacturers. Over the past 10 years she has received a salary from Rutgers University, with research funding support from the N.J. Department of Health, the Research Foundation for Mental Hygiene/Columbia University Center for Practice Innovation, and the National Institutes of Health. She also has been a consultant to the American Lung Association. She has no additional information to disclose.

Jonathan Foulds has done paid consulting for J&J on clinical trial design in the past 3 years. Prior to that he has done paid consulting for pharmaceutical companies involved in producing smoking cessation medications, including GSK, Pfizer, Novartis, J&J, and Cypress Bioscience, and he received a research grant from Pfizer. He has in the past acted as an expert witness (for plaintiffs) in litigation against tobacco companies. He has not done any paid work for tobacco or electronic cigarette manufacturers. Over the past 10 years he has received a salary from Penn State University, and his research has been continuously funded by the National Institutes of Health.

Acknowledgments

We would like to thank all of the people who made our careers in tobacco treatment and research possible. In particular, we would like to thank those who were mentors and influential in our field but are no longer with us, particularly Drs. John Slade, Michael Russell, and John Hughes.

We would also like to thank our friends, colleagues, and family members who put up with our perhaps overly extensive discussions about nicotine addiction over the years. Thanks for your patience and support.

Finally, we would like to thank the many patients and research participants who took the time to tell us why they smoked, why they wanted to quit, what helped, and why it was not as easy as some may think. Without their insights, this book would not have been written.

Foreword

Cigarette smoking remains one of the most important causes of premature morbidity and mortality. Smoking causes premature cardiovascular disease, chronic lung disease, cancer, increased susceptibility to and severity of respiratory tract infection, and other disease, resulting in an average 10 years of life lost in someone who smokes lifelong. Quitting smoking at any age substantially reduces the risk of disease and improves longevity.

Although the prevalence of smoking in developed countries has declined in recent years, smoking rates in subsets of the population, particularly people with mental illness and substance use disorders and those who are financially disadvantaged, remain high. Smoking cessation is a critical goal of public health and should be a priority in all medical care settings.

Cigarette smoking and the use of other tobacco products is driven by addiction to nicotine. Nicotine addiction results in changes in the structure and function of the brain. People who smoke consume nicotine to modulate mood and arousal, and for pleasure, and experience withdrawal symptoms when they do not have nicotine. Many consume nicotine to cope with stress and other challenges in daily life, making quitting difficult.

Drs. Jill Williams and Jonathan Foulds address the challenges of smoking cessation in *Treating Addiction to Tobacco and Nicotine Products*. They review the range of treatments, including various behavioral interventions, pharmacotherapies, and the use of non-combusted nicotine products, such as electronic (e-)cigarettes. The use of such products is viewed within a continuum of risk of nicotine products, with combusted nicotine products being most harmful and non-combusted products being able to address the need for nicotine in a less harmful way. This book examines the benefits and risks of such products in promoting smoking cessation.

Most important, this book examines management of nicotine addiction in clinical settings, including in people with mental health and substance use disorders. Clinical vignettes are presented, followed by discussion of management approaches, which will be of particular interest to clinicians. This book provides excellent guidance for health professionals who are treating tobacco addiction, the success of which will save many lives.

Neal L. Benowitz, M.D.
Professor of Medicine, University of California, San Francisco
Former President of the Society for Research on Nicotine and Tobacco

Preface

Tobacco use continues to be the leading preventable cause of death in our country, especially affecting people with mental illness. Addiction psychiatry and partners from many other disciplines have worked hard and produced groundbreaking advances in the assessment and treatment of people who use tobacco and nicotine products. Today, we have safe and highly effective pharmacological treatments and powerful psychosocial approaches to help people with smoking cessation. However, access to these lifesaving interventions continues to be hampered by complex societal, cultural, and economic barriers.

In addition, electronic cigarettes and vaping have added another layer of complexity to our work. On one hand, evidence is growing in terms of vaping helping adults quit smoking. On the other hand, people who have never smoked cigarettes, particularly young people, can become addicted and incur health problems by vaping.

This comprehensive, balanced, and thoroughly up-to-date book is an invaluable tool for psychiatrists and other clinicians in our everyday work caring for people who smoke and vape. Furthermore, it will also educate parents, students, school counselors, employee assistance counselors, judges, journalists, academics, and politicians about the latest advances in the treatment of addiction to tobacco and nicotine products and help our communities thrive.

Petros Levounis, M.D., M.A.
Immediate Past President, American Psychiatric Association,
Washington, D.C.; Professor and Chair, Department of Psychiatry
Associate Dean, Rutgers New Jersey Medical School, Newark,
New Jersey

Introduction

Seismic changes are underway in the worldwide use of nicotine and tobacco. Decades of declining cigarette use rates in the United States since the 1964 landmark report from the Surgeon General seemed to suggest this problem was on its way to being solved. However, ongoing high rates of cigarette smoking among people with less education or poor mental health, as well as the emergence of new products and methods of nicotine delivery, mean that tobacco use continues to be a major public health and clinical challenge. Clean indoor air policies, advertising restrictions, public health education campaigns, access to effective treatments, and increased taxes are all effective at changing the perception of smoking and driving tobacco use down. In many countries, smoking rates have fallen, and the proportion of U.S. adults who smoke cigarettes continues to decline, dropping from around 15% in 2015 to 11% in 2023. Despite this success, vulnerable subpopulations, such as those with co-occurring behavioral health conditions, could be left behind, with tobacco use rates two to three times higher than in the general population. Only in the past decade have important tobacco control organizations started to make this group a priority, and this increased recognition will be essential for bringing these individuals needed resources and treatment strategies.

Even with reduced smoking rates, tobacco smoking remains one of the main causes of preventable death and disease in the United States and in most countries of the world. On average, people who smoke long-term die 10 years earlier than people who do not smoke. Tobacco causes a staggering 50% of deaths among people with serious mental illness and kills more substance users than their primary substance of use. Tobacco also threatens recovery by negatively impacting finances, employability, housing, mental health symptoms, and abstinence from other substances.

At the same time that the use of cigarettes is declining, the use of other nicotine and tobacco products is stable or increasing, requiring surveillance of a widening variety of products whose risks have not been fully determined. The emergence of new nicotine products, including heated tobacco products and nicotine pouches that contain no tobacco, has also dramatically changed the tobacco control landscape. Indeed, the end of cigarettes may be on the horizon as the tobacco industry recognizes the increasing popularity of these innovative, non-combustible products. Serious questions remain, however, about the safety of these products for long-term use because regulatory agencies are only beginning to evaluate the scientific evidence.

Of great concern always is the impact on young people and the potential of nicotine exposure to influence brain development and vulnerability for addiction. The rapid rise in electronic (e-)cigarette use and vaping among teens and young adults in the past decade is a serious cause for concern. The use of flavors and advertising that appeal to young people clearly requires more regulation. The safety and efficacy of e-cigarettes as an aid to cessation is subject to debate, but there is now strong evidence that this is a viable strategy for some adults who smoke cigarettes. Nicotine delivery from some of these new products can be similar to that from cigarettes, suggesting that although toxicant exposure is reduced, addiction to nicotine will often continue. Effective treatments for quitting e-cigarettes and other nicotine-containing products are only beginning to be studied rigorously.

There is overwhelming evidence that quitting cigarette use saves lives and is beneficial to health at any age. Effective treatments exist for tobacco use disorder (TUD), yet half of people who saw a health professional in the past year did not receive advice to quit smoking, and most adults who smoke do not use evidence-based treatment (VanFrank et al. 2024). This may be worse in mental health settings, where less than half of providers *even ask* their patients about smoking. There are also marked disparities in cessation behaviors (past-year quit attempt and cessation) by educational level, poverty, age, health insurance, race/ethnicity, and geography. Most people who smoke want to quit completely. Treatments are safe and effective, yet vastly underutilized.

There is clearly a need for health care professionals to provide more evidence-based therapies for TUD; this is particularly true in behavioral health settings, where tobacco treatment has not been a priority. Removing barriers to accessing tobacco dependence treatment by increasing treatment capacity is essential in all health care settings. Because smoking is becoming more concentrated in vulnerable populations, there is a need for approaches that are inclusive, are culturally sensitive, and address these barriers. Although live and online training programs exist, few recent books have focused on the scientific basis and comprehensive clinical skills needed for treating tobacco addiction, particularly since the recent increase in availability of non-smoked nicotine products.

To that end, we created this comprehensive and up-to-date book focused on the assessment and treatment of TUD that we hope will be an essential resource for a wide range of health care professionals because tobacco use impacts all aspects of health care. We include sections on trends in tobacco use, including new products such as e-cigarettes, the biology of nicotine addiction, and strategies for changing health care systems. The book is designed for the busy clinician and is a synthesis of current literature and best practices. In places where evidence is lacking, we apply clinical judgment and experience with other addictions. We include case vignettes and summarize key points at the end of each chapter. Recognizing the high rates of tobacco use among individuals with mental health and other substance use problems, we have attempted to make the book particularly relevant for clinicians who care for those populations.

Initial chapters review current trends in the use of tobacco and other emerging products. Chapter 1 is an up-to-date review of the harms from cigarette smoke and other tobacco products. Chapter 2 discusses how the pattern of use of nicotine products has changed and includes a broad range of products, including combustible (e.g., cigarettes, cigars) and non-combustible (e.g., e-cigarettes) products. Although it is not easy to compare all potential long-term harms of traditional and novel nicotine products with precision, there is widespread consensus that smoked products (particularly cigarettes) are likely significantly more harmful than non-smoked nicotine products. The use of non-cigarette and non-smoked nicotine products likely will continue to gain market share, and "dual use" of cigarettes and other products likely will continue to increase as more nicotine products are developed and as the scientific evidence on their risks and benefits develops.

Chapter 3 discusses the neurobiology of TUD, the DSM-5 (American Psychiatric Association 2022) criteria for the disorder, and tobacco withdrawal symptoms. Chapter 4 discusses clinical approaches to TUD and how to conduct assessments. When assessing nicotine addiction, it is important to ask about the use of *any* nicotine products, not just cigarettes or the product the person uses most frequently. Chapter 5 provides a review of tobacco comorbidity with other behavioral health conditions, including epidemiology and a review of unique consequences experienced by people with these comorbidities.

The remainder of the book (Chapters 6–12) focuses on clinical treatment approaches, with chapters on evidence-based counseling and pharmacotherapy. Chapter 6 reviews the solid evidence that obtaining behavioral support can increase the chances of successfully quitting smoking. Patients who smoke should be informed about the behavioral support options that are available, and it should be made clear to them that there is good evidence these treatments help participants to quit. Chapter 7 reviews the use of pharmacotherapy treatments. Medications are a first-line treatment with a large evidence base demonstrating safety and efficacy. Most people do not use these medications correctly, in a high enough dosage, or for a long enough time, which undermines success in a quit attempt. We also discuss special populations for whom the evidence is limited; in these instances, clinical judgment should err on the side of providing treatment whenever possible because the continued risks of smoking are nearly always worse than the potential risk from the specific treatment. We also discuss emerging treatments such as cytisine and transcranial magnetic stimulation in Chapter 7.

In Chapter 8, we include approaches for counseling patients who may not be immediately ready to quit smoking. Every tobacco user should receive treatment of some kind, with an emphasis on engaging people in strategies to change. Sustaining behavior change can be challenging, and Chapter 9 discusses strategies for preventing a return to smoking and creating a tobacco-free lifestyle. Chapter 10 reviews how changes made at the systems level can help to implement more widespread or systematic change by supporting the clinical interventions of individual health care providers. Promoting health systems change is effective in reducing the number of people using tobacco by institutionalizing prevention and treatment interventions in health care settings and integrating these into routine clinic care.

Chapter 11 highlights clinical issues in the treatment of TUD in people with mental illness and other substance use. Many studies have demonstrated that trying to quit smoking does not worsen mental illness, although this can be complicated in the short term by tobacco withdrawal symptoms that mimic symptoms of mental illness. Illness severity and functional impairment may ultimately be more important prognostic factors than discrete diagnostic subgroups, although some subgroups such as those with depression or schizophrenia are reviewed. The tobacco and nicotine marketplace is currently shifting away from smoked products toward the use of non-smoked nicotine products, and Chapter 12 reviews the potential benefits of making this switch. A consideration is that non-smoked products (e.g., e-cigarettes, snus, nicotine pouches, heat-not-burn cigarettes) all deliver nicotine and therefore can be addictive. This chapter also includes discussion of helping non-cigarette tobacco users to quit.

References

American Psychiatric Association: Diagnostic and Statistical Manual of Mental Disorders, 5th Edition, Text Revision. Washington, DC, American Psychiatric Association, 2022

VanFrank B, Malarcher A, Cornelius ME, et al: Adult Smoking Cessation—United States, 2022. MMWR Morb Mortal Wkly Rep 73:633–641, 2024

1

Trends in and Harms From Cigarette Smoking

Since the invention of the cigarette-making machine toward the end of the nineteenth century and then throughout the twentieth century, cigarettes have been by far the most common form of nicotine consumed in the United States, with cigars and oral tobacco (chew and snuff) trailing far behind. Despite declines in use, smoking remains the number-one cause of preventable death in the United States, where it has been estimated to cause more than 400,000 premature deaths per year (Thun et al. 2000). Tobacco smoking also causes more than 4.9 million deaths per year worldwide (8.8% of all global deaths) (World Health Organization 1997). Even as the proportion of U.S. adults who smoke cigarettes continues to decline, important disparities in cigarette smoking persist, and tobacco use remains strongly linked to socioeconomic status. Higher rates also are consistently seen in populations with behavioral health comorbidity.

Changes in Prevalence

At the time of the landmark 1964 U.S. Surgeon General's report on tobacco and health, more than 50% of men and 30% of women smoked cigarettes (Centers for Disease Control and Prevention 1999). That report concluded that cigarettes were a cause of lung cancer, and numerous follow-up reports clarified the enormous harmfulness of cigarette smoking.

1

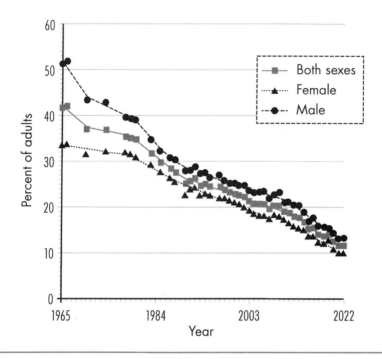

Figure 1–1. Decline in U.S. adult male and female cigarette smoking prevalence, 1965–2022.

Source. Reprinted from National Cancer Institute: "Adult Tobacco Use," in *Cancer Trends Progress Report.* Bethesda, MD, National Cancer Institute, March 2024. Available at: https://progressreport.cancer.gov. Accessed June 25, 2024.

Substantial public health efforts over the following decades (including education about the health effects, increased cigarette taxes, smoke-free air legislation, and establishment of age-of-sale laws) succeeded in consistently reducing the prevalence of cigarette smoking such that, by 2020, only 14% of men and 11% of women smoked cigarettes "every day or some days" (Cornelius et al. 2022; Wang et al. 2018). This decline in prevalence among the sexes in the United States (shown in Figure 1–1) has been gradual and might have been expected to have occurred much more quickly. However, over the latter half of the twentieth century, the tobacco industry mounted an aggressive public relations campaign to sow seeds of doubt about this scientific evidence, despite themselves knowing the addictive and harmful nature of tobacco.

In 1963, Addison Yeaman, then executive vice president of Brown and Williamson Tobacco Corporation and president of the Committee for Tobacco Research, wrote:

> Moreover, nicotine is addictive. We are, then, in the business of sell-
> ing nicotine, an addictive drug....But cigarettes...despite the benefi-
> cent effect of nicotine, have certain unattractive side effects: 1) They
> cause, or predispose to, lung cancer. 2) They contribute to certain car-
> diovascular disorders. 3) They may well be truly causative in emphy-
> sema....(Slade et al. 1995)

As recently as 1998, Philip Morris chairman Geoffrey Bible responded to the question *"Has* anyone died from smoking cigarettes?" in the fol-lowing manner: "I don't know if anyone dies from smoking tobacco, I just don't know" (Geyelin 1998). While cigarettes remain by far the most commonly used tobacco or nicotine product in the United States, since the beginning of the twenty-first century the tobacco industry has increasingly acknowledged the scientific consensus on the addic-tiveness and other health effects of cigarettes and has diversified into marketing a range of other products. Among U.S. adults in 2020, 12.5% smoked cigarettes, 3.7% used electronic (e-)cigarettes, 3.5% smoked cigars, and 2.3% used smokeless tobacco products (Cornelius et al. 2022). In addition, tobacco smoked in hookahs, a form of tobacco tra-ditionally used in the Middle East, has become popular among U.S. college students. More recently, the industry has developed and started marketing other products, such as "heat-not-burn" cigarettes and tobacco-free nicotine pouches, small tea bag–like sachets containing a white powder with nicotine, flavors, and sweeteners but no tobacco (Sparrock et al. 2023).

Because cigarettes continue to be by far the most commonly used tobacco product, for most of this chapter we focus on describing the harms to health from smoking cigarettes. In later chapters (see Chapters 2, 4, and 12), we cover the relative harms from other products.

Diseases Caused by Cigarette Smoking

Numerous reviews of the scientific evidence on the health effects of smoking have shown that cigarette smoking harms almost every part of the human body. Table 1–1 lists some of the deadly diseases known to be caused by tobacco smoking, along with the relative risks of death from each cause in people who continue to smoke or who previously smoked compared with people who never smoked. In all of these diseases, the evidence was judged sufficient to infer a causal relationship rather than a noncausal association. What Table 1–1 shows is that men who continue to smoke throughout their life are 10.9 times more likely to die from cancer of the lip, oral cavity, or pharynx than those who never smoked. The highest relative risk, not surprisingly, is for cancer of the trachea, bronchus, and lung, from which men who continue to smoke are 23.3 times more likely to die than those who never smoked.

Smoking is also the established cause of a number of other nonfatal diseases and conditions, including cataracts, periodontitis, acute respiratory infections in people with chronic obstructive pulmonary disease (COPD), acute respiratory symptoms in adults and children (e.g., coughing and wheezing), adverse surgical outcomes related to wound healing and respiratory complications, and hip fractures (Office of the Surgeon General 2004).

Tobacco smoking has been estimated to cause more than 400,000 premature deaths per year in the United States (Thun et al. 2000) and 4.9 million deaths per year worldwide (8.8% of all global deaths) (World Health Organization 1997). In developed countries, most of these deaths are from cardiovascular diseases, followed by cancer (predominantly of the lung) and then COPD. Tobacco smoking causes more premature deaths each year in the United States than alcohol, illegal drugs, AIDS, road traffic accidents, homicide, and suicide combined (McGinnis and Foege 1993), and every year it causes premature deaths in the United States at a rate comparable with those caused per year by coronavirus disease 2019 (COVID-19) during the period from 2020 to 2022 (Foulds et al. 2023). For every case of premature death caused by tobacco smoking each year in the United States, approximately 20 cases of nonfatal serious smoking-caused illnesses are diagnosed. The vast majority of these illnesses (59%) are chronic respiratory diseases (e.g., COPD) (Centers for Disease Control and Prevention 2003). The net effect of these smoking-caused diseases is that the person who continues to smoke is likely to die an average of 10 years earlier than someone who never smoked (Doll et al. 2004). The approximate doubling of mortality risks for people who smoke is evident at age 50 (6% have already died vs. 3% of people who never smoked) and continues past age 70 (by which age 42% have died vs. 19%).

Table 1–1. Cancer Prevention Study (CPS-II) age-adjusted relative risk of death from smoking-related diseases for people who continue to smoke or formerly smoked compared with those who never smoked

| | CPS-II (1982–1988) | | | |
| | Men | | Women | |
Disease category	Continue to smoke	Formerly smoked	Continue to smoke	Formerly smoked
Neoplasms				
Lip, oral cavity, pharynx	10.9	3.4	5.1	2.3
Esophagus	6.8	4.5	7.8	2.8
Stomach	2	1.5	1.4	1.3
Pancreas	2.3	1.2	2.3	1.6
Larynx	14.6	6.3	13	5.2
Trachea, bronchus, lung	23.3	8.7	12.7	4.5
Cervix uteri			1.6	1.1
Urinary bladder	3.3	2.1	2.2	1.9
Kidney, other urinary	2.7	1.7	1.3	1.1
Acute myeloid leukemia	1.9	1.3	1.1	1.4

Table 1–1. Cancer Prevention Study (CPS-II) age-adjusted relative risk of death from smoking-related diseases for people who continue to smoke or formerly smoked compared with those who never smoked (*continued*)

| Disease category | CPS-II (1982–1988) | | | |
| | Men | | Women | |
	Continue to smoke	Formerly smoked	Continue to smoke	Formerly smoked
Cardiovascular diseases				
Ischemic heart disease				
Ages 35–64 years	2.8	1.6	3.1	1.3
Age ≥65 years	1.5	1.2	1.6	1.2
Other heart disease	1.8	1.2	1.5	1.1
Cerebrovascular disease				
Ages 35–64 years	3.3	1	4	1.3
Age ≥65 years	1.6	1	1.5	1
Atherosclerosis	2.4	1.3	1.8	1
Aortic aneurysm	6.2	3.1	7.1	2.1
Other arterial disease	2.1	1	2.2	1.1

Table 1–1. Cancer Prevention Study (CPS-II) age-adjusted relative risk of death from smoking-related diseases for people who continue to smoke or formerly smoked compared with those who never smoked (*continued*)

	CPS-II (1982–1988)			
	Men		Women	
Disease category	Continue to smoke	Formerly smoked	Continue to smoke	Formerly smoked
Respiratory diseases				
Pneumonia, influenza	1.8	1.4	2.2	1.1
Bronchitis, emphysema	17.1	15.6	12	11.8
Chronic airways obstruction	10.6	6.8	13.1	6.8
Perinatal conditions				
Short gestation/low birth weight			1.8	
Respiratory distress syndrome			1.3	
Other respiratory conditions			1.4	
Sudden infant death syndrome			2.3	

Note. A relative risk of 1 implies no increased risk in people who smoke/have smoked, and a relative risk of 2 implies a doubling of the risk of death due to that disease in people who smoke/have smoked compared with people who never smoked.

Source. Adapted from Office of the Surgeon General 2004, Table 7–1.1.

Dose-Response Relationship Between Cigarette Smoking and Disease

For most of the smoking-caused diseases just mentioned, there is also evidence of a significant dose-response relationship between the total amount of smoking and the risk of contracting the disease. The most striking dose-response relationship is typically found in lung cancer, as shown in Table 1–1. However, reductions in some disease and mortality risks tend to be disappointingly small or nonexistent when people who smoke reduce their cigarette consumption per day (Godtfredsen et al. 2002). This is likely because they "compensate" by inhaling more from each cigarette to obtain their preferred dose of nicotine (Benowitz et al. 1986). It has also been established that the duration of smoking (i.e., number of years smoking) is a much larger determinant of some disease risks (e.g., lung cancer) than the number of cigarettes smoked per day (Knoke et al. 2004). Thus, many epidemiological studies use the term *pack years* (packs of cigarettes per day multiplied by number of years smoking) as a crude measure of smoking dose, and this measure is often significantly related to disease risk.

Although age itself is frequently a potent predictor of the risk of many of the smoking-caused diseases, nonetheless it is clear that the earlier a person quits smoking, the lower their risk of disease, independent of their age. For example, a person who never smoked has a cumulative risk of death from lung cancer by age 75 of less than 0.5%, whereas someone who continues to smoke to age 75 has a 16% cumulative risk and a person who quit smoking by age 50 has a 6% cumulative risk (Peto et al. 2000). The 2020 U.S. Surgeon General's report reviewed the health benefits of ceasing tobacco use and concluded that smoking cessation has major health benefits for people of all ages. For example, those who quit smoking by age 50 have half the risk of dying over the next 15 years compared with those who continue to smoke (United States Public Health Service Office of the Surgeon General and National Center for Chronic Disease Prevention and Health Promotion [US] Office on Smoking and Health 2020). The time scale for reduction in risks of disease after smoking cessation varies with each disease and even with the stage of the disease. Thus, the excess risk of death from coronary heart disease is cut in half within 1 year of stopping smoking, but the same level of risk reduction for lung cancer may take 10–15 years (United States Public Health Service Office of the Surgeon General and

National Center for Chronic Disease Prevention and Health Promotion [US] Office on Smoking and Health 2020).

Lung function declines with age after reaching adulthood in people who never smoked, but it declines at a significantly faster rate for people who smoke. However, when someone stops smoking, they typically have an absolute improvement in lung function within 1 year of stopping, and then their rate of lung function decline normalizes to a rate similar to that of those who never smoked (Scanlon et al. 2000).

Toxicants in Cigarette Smoke and Their Relationship to Disease Causation

Cigarettes typically contain a large number of ingredients, including the tobacco leaf, tobacco paper, filter (fibers of which may be inhaled) (Pauly et al. 2002), and more than 500 potential additives (e.g., acetaldehyde, ammonia, cocoa, levulinic acid, menthol). When the cigarette is lit and the tip burns, it reaches extremely high temperatures (>400°C), rising to more than 600°C as air is sucked into the cone (White et al. 2001). The resulting smoke is composed of a complex mixture of more than 4,000 chemicals resulting from pyrolysis. Many of these chemicals exist in very small quantities just above the detection limits of sensitive toxicology assays, but many highly toxic chemicals are present in large measurable concentrations in tobacco smoke and are known to be involved in causing various diseases. Table 1–2 provides examples of some of the main classes of toxicants in tobacco smoke from the FDA's list of 93 harmful and potentially harmful constituents (Cheng et al. 2022).

Many of the mechanisms whereby this complex mixture of toxicants in tobacco smoke lead to specific diseases have been identified. For example, a large number of these chemicals have been shown to cause cancer in animals or humans (e.g., benzo[a]pyrene, 4-[methylnitrosamino]-1-[3-pyridyl]-1-butanone [NNK], and *N*-nitrosonornicotine [NNN]). These chemicals cause DNA damage, inflammation, and oxidative stress, which promote the initiation and growth of tumors (Hecht 1999). The deposition of tar particles in the lungs and upper airways leads to their blockage and to COPD. The toxic chemicals stimulate oxidative stress, inflammation, and a reduction in elastin, inhibiting the elasticity of the lungs and hence the ability to inhale and exhale normally. Irritants such as nitric oxide cause hypersecretion of mucus, and substances such as acrolein, acetone, and acetaldehyde damage the cilia (inhibiting its

Table 1–2. Examples of toxicants in tobacco smoke (from more than 7,000 identified chemicals)

Volatile organic substances	Polycyclic aromatic hydrocarbons
1,3-Butadiene (RT, RDT)	Benzo(a)pyrene (CA)
Benzene (CA, CT, RDT)	Pyrene (CA)
Toluene (RT, RDT)	Benz(a)anthracene (CA, CT)
Gaseous substances	**Nitrosamines**
Ammonia (RT)	N-nitrosonornicotine (NNN) (CA)
Hydrogen cyanide (RT, CT)	4-(Methylnitrosamino)-1-(3-pyridyl)-1-butanone (NNK) (CA)
Carbon monoxide (RDT)	N-nitrosodimethylamine (CA)
Metals	**Carbonyls**
Lead (CA, CT, RDT)	Formaldehyde (CA, RT)
Cadmium (CA, RT, RDT)	Acetaldehyde (CA, RT, AD)
Arsenic (CA, CT, RDT)	Acrolein (RT, CT)
Aromatic amines	**Aza-arenes**
4-Aminobiphenyl (CA)	Quinoline (CA)
1-Aminonaphthalene (CA)	IQ (2-amino-3-methylimidazo[4,5-*f*] quinoline) (CA)

Note. Each of these examples is on the list of 93 chemicals and chemical compounds identified by the FDA as harmful and potentially harmful constituents in tobacco products and tobacco smoke as required by the Food, Drug, and Cosmetic Act. The letters after each chemical name indicate the main types of toxic effects known for each chemical as follows: carcinogen (CA), respiratory toxicant (RT), cardiovascular toxicant (CT), reproductive or developmental toxicant (RDT), addictive (AD).

ability to clear mucus), which also contributes to chronic decrements in respiratory function. Years of smoking and daily coating of the lungs and airways in tar lead to irreversible lung damage and ultimately to death from COPD.

The carbon monoxide in smoke replaces oxygen in the hemoglobin, adversely affecting oxygen transport and energy supply and requiring the heart to do more work to supply the same amount of oxygen to the body. A large number of smoke constituents, and particularly the volatile components of the gaseous phase of tobacco smoke, cause oxidative stress, immunological responses, and inflammation in the endothelial cells (Powell 1998). The resultant platelet aggregation, plaque formation, and inhibition of vasorelaxation contribute to endothelial malfunction and thrombosis. These processes increase the likelihood of myocardial infarction, stroke, or other cardiovascular problems. Acute nicotine administration increases heart rate and blood pressure and causes peripheral vasoconstriction (i.e., impairs peripheral circulation, thus exacerbating Raynaud's disease and erectile dysfunction). However, studies of smokeless tobacco users (who also have high nicotine exposure but without the smoke) compared with people who smoke suggest that most cardiovascular problems are not caused by nicotine. For example, smoking, but not snuff use, is associated with peripheral artery disease (Yuan et al. 2022), and snuff users have consistently been found to have lower risks of myocardial infarction than people who smoke (Yuan et al. 2022). It therefore appears that the thrombogenic effects of tobacco smoke exposure (primarily oxidant gases)—combined with reduced oxygen supply (carbon monoxide) and increased myocardial oxygen demand (nicotine)—are the cause of cardiovascular harm from smoking (Office of the Surgeon General 2004).

What should be clear from this discussion is that inhalation into the lungs of tobacco smoke containing thousands of toxicants is the primary reason cigarette smoking is so extremely harmful to health. Inhalation of smoke from other combusted forms of tobacco (e.g., cigars, hookah) is harmful through similar mechanisms, but their overall harms largely depend on a combination of the amount of smoke toxicants inhaled per day and the number of years these products are used in this manner. The frequency and duration of use are therefore major determinants of the long-term harms that will result and are influenced in part by how addictive or dependence-forming the product is. The addictiveness of cigarettes and other nicotine products is discussed in more detail in subsequent chapters (see Chapters 2, 3, 4, and 12), but it should be evident, given their continued widespread and long duration of use despite widely recognized harms, that cigarettes are the most addictive form of nicotine consumption yet developed.

Harms From Exposure to Environmental Tobacco Smoke

Despite continued counterclaims from the tobacco industry, environmental tobacco smoke (ETS) has emerged as a major preventable health

Table 1–3. Effects causally associated with exposure to environmental tobacco smoke

Developmental effects

Low birthweight

Sudden infant death syndrome (SIDS)

Preterm delivery

Respiratory effects

Acute lower respiratory tract infections in children (e.g., bronchitis and pneumonia)

Asthma induction and exacerbation in children and adults

Chronic respiratory symptoms in children

Middle ear infections in children

Carcinogenic effects

Lung cancer

Nasal sinus cancer

Breast cancer in younger, primarily premenopausal females

Cardiovascular effects

Coronary artery disease

hazard in our society. As with other major pollutants, ETS exposure is often involuntary and frequently unavoidable. Because tobacco smoke is one of the most potent toxic compounds, ETS pollution can impact many health problems, even with low levels of exposure (Prignot 2011). Table 1–3 lists some of the most common health effects that have been causally linked to ETS.

The evidence currently available demonstrates that ETS exposure poses a serious public health problem, and policies designed to protect the public from secondhand smoke must be continued in order to limit its deadly impact. Such policies can lead to specific clinical management requirements for people who smoke tobacco but who find themselves living or working in an institutional environment such as a hospital, psychiatric unit, or prison where smoking is banned indoors (Ratschen et al. 2009).

Changes in Patterns of Cigarette Use

One of the major public health success stories of the twenty-first century in the United States has been the marked reduction in cigarette smoking among schoolchildren (Sun et al. 2021). Perhaps the best-quality data on this have been produced by the Monitoring the Future project at the University of Michigan, where large representative surveys have been conducted of substance use and other health risk factors among schoolchildren since 1976 (Johnston et al. 2019). As shown in Figure 1–2, past-30-day cigarette smoking was more than 36% among U.S. twelfth-grade students as recently as 1997 but has declined substantially since then to 4.1% in 2021, with only 2% of twelfth graders smoking daily, compared with 24.6% in 1997.

Recent evidence suggests that these gains in youth cigarette smoking are being maintained among the 18- to 24-year-old age group. Studies of smoking cessation found that rates of annual smoking cessation among adults who smoked increased by more than 4.2% during the period from 2008 to 2013 and 5.4% from 2014 to 2019. With current initiation and cessation rates, smoking prevalence should fall to 8.3% in 2030 and eventually reach a steady state of 3.5% (Méndez et al. 2022). Even in recent decades, as the proportion of U.S. adults who smoke cigarettes continues to decline, important disparities in cigarette smoking persist, and tobacco use remains strongly linked to socioeconomic status. Cigarette smoking rates are higher among men, Native Americans, and groups with less education, with low income, or who were uninsured or insured through Medicaid (Jamal et al. 2018). Much higher tobacco use rates are also seen among military veterans, individuals with a disability, or people who identify as lesbian, gay, or bisexual (Odani et al. 2018). As of 2020, more than 30 million U.S. adults currently smoked cigarettes, and cigarette smoking was markedly more prevalent among people with co-occurring mental disorders or substance use disorders (Cornelius et al. 2022; Prochaska et al. 2017). Rates of smoking among people with a behavioral health condition are at least double the rates seen in the general population (Smith et al. 2014). Evidence shows that smoking rates are not declining as rapidly among these disparate groups (Cook et al. 2014), suggesting that smoking will become increasingly concentrated in these populations if more is not done to prevent it.

For most people who smoke, the single most important thing they can do to improve their health is to quit smoking, and one of the most

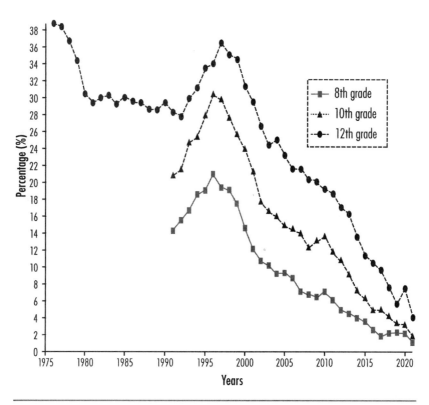

Figure 1–2. Percentage of U.S. eighth-, tenth-, and twelfth-grade students who have smoked at least one cigarette in the previous 30 days, as assessed in the Monitoring the Future study, 1975–2021.
Source.   Reprinted from Miech RA, Johnston LD, O'Malley PM, et al: *Monitoring the Future National Survey Results on Drug Use, 1975–2021, Vol I: Secondary School Students.* Ann Arbor, MI, Institute for Social Research, University of Michigan, 2023. Available at: https://monitoringthefuture.org/wp-content/uploads /2022/12/mtf2022.pdf. Accessed August 4, 2024.

important interventions a clinician can make is to help a patient succeed in quitting.

Case Example

During the first meeting of a smoking cessation support group, we were going around the group as people introduced themselves and expressed why they wanted to quit. Janice stated that she had been smoking for more than 35 years, her breathing had become more difficult, and she had recently been diagnosed with COPD. Her doctor told her she had to quit or her breathing would worsen rapidly, and that was why she was now attending the group. Next was George, a 62-year-old man who said proudly that he had been smoking for 50 years, since he was 12 years old. "But I'm not like Janice; smoking hasn't made me seriously ill yet, touch wood. I did have a heart attack 2 years ago and surgery on the veins in my legs a few years before that, but so far, my lungs are okay!" When asked whether he had been told that cigarette smoking causes peripheral vascular disease and heart attacks, George said no and that he thought smoking only caused lung problems, because that was where the smoke goes.

What Are the Concerns in This Case?

Although more than 90% of people who smoke are aware that it causes lung cancer, far fewer are aware that smoking causes all the other diseases listed in Table 1–1 and many more. So whenever the opportunity presents itself, it is worth checking that the patient understands that a disease they have, or that they have a family history of, is worsened by smoking and that their risks may be reduced by quitting completely.

Key Points

- Smoke from a burning cigarette contains more than 4,000 chemicals.
- Cigarette smoking harms almost every part of the human body.
- The earlier a person quits smoking, the greater their reduction in smoking-attributable disease risk.
- The toxicity from tobacco smoke is so high that even passive exposure to tobacco smoke pollution can increase the risks for numerous diseases.

References

Benowitz NL, Jacob P III, Kozlowski LT, et al: Influence of smoking fewer cigarettes on exposure to tar, nicotine, and carbon monoxide. N Engl J Med 315(21):1310–1313, 1986 3773954

Centers for Disease Control and Prevention: Tobacco use—United States, 1900–1999. MMWR Morb Mortal Wkly Rep 48(43):986–993, 1999 10577492

Centers for Disease Control and Prevention: Cigarette smoking-attributable morbidity—United States, 2000. MMWR Morb Mortal Wkly Rep 52(35):842–844, 2003 12966360

Cheng T, Reilly SM, Feng C, et al: Harmful and potentially harmful constituents in the filler and smoke of tobacco-containing tobacco products. ACS Omega 7(29):25537–25554, 2022 35910156

Cook BL, Wayne GF, Kafali EN, et al: Trends in smoking among adults with mental illness and association between mental health treatment and smoking cessation. JAMA 311(2):172–182, 2014 24399556

Cornelius ME, Loretan CG, Wang TW, et al: Tobacco product use among adults—United States, 2020. MMWR Morb Mortal Wkly Rep 71(11):397–405, 2022 35298455

Doll R, Peto R, Boreham J, et al: Mortality in relation to smoking: 50 years' observations on male British doctors. BMJ 328(7455):1519, 2004 15213107

Foulds J, Allen SI, Yingst J: Cytisinicline to speed smoking cessation in the United States. JAMA 330(2):129–130, 2023 37432430

Geyelin M: Tobacco executive doubts product risks. Wall Street Journal, March 3, 1998

Godtfredsen NS, Holst C, Prescott E, et al: Smoking reduction, smoking cessation, and mortality: a 16-year follow-up of 19,732 men and women from The Copenhagen Centre for Prospective Population Studies. Am J Epidemiol 156(11):994–1001, 2002 12446255

Hecht SS: Tobacco smoke carcinogens and lung cancer. J Natl Cancer Inst 91(14):1194–1210, 1999 10413421

Jamal A, Phillips E, Gentzke AS, et al: Current cigarette smoking among adults—United States, 2016. MMWR Morb Mortal Wkly Rep 67(2):53–59, 2018 29346338

Johnston LD, Miech RA, O'Malley PM, et al: Monitoring the Future National Survey Results on Drug Use 1975–2018: Overview, Key Findings on Adolescent Drug Use. Ann Arbor, MI, University of Michigan Institute for Social Research, 2019

Knoke JD, Shanks TG, Vaughn JW, et al: Lung cancer mortality is related to age in addition to duration and intensity of cigarette smoking: an analysis of CPS-I data. Cancer Epidemiol Biomarkers Prev 13(6):949–957, 2004 15184251

McGinnis JM, Foege WH: Actual causes of death in the United States. JAMA 270(18):2207–2212, 1993 8411605

Méndez D, Le TTT, Warner KE: Monitoring the increase in the U.S. smoking cessation rate and its implication for future smoking prevalence. Nicotine Tob Res 24(11):1727–1731, 2022 35486922

Odani S, Agaku IT, Graffunder CM, et al: Tobacco product use among military veterans—United States, 2010–2015. MMWR Morb Mortal Wkly Rep 67(1):7–12, 2018 29324732

Office of the Surgeon General: The Health Consequences of Smoking: A Report of the Surgeon General. Atlanta, GA, Centers for Disease Control and Prevention, 2004. Available at: https://www.ncbi.nlm.nih.gov/books/NBK44695. Accessed August 4, 2024.

Pauly JL, Mepani AB, Lesses JD, et al: Cigarettes with defective filters marketed for 40 years: what Philip Morris never told smokers. Tob Control 11(Suppl 1):I51–I61, 2002

Peto R, Darby S, Deo H, et al: Smoking, smoking cessation, and lung cancer in the UK since 1950: combination of national statistics with two case-control studies. BMJ 321(7257):323–329, 2000 10926586

Powell JT: Vascular damage from smoking: disease mechanisms at the arterial wall. Vasc Med 3(1):21–28, 1998 9666528

Prignot JJ: Recent contributions of air- and biomarkers to the control of secondhand smoke (SHS): a review. Int J Environ Res Public Health 8(3):648–682, 2011 21556172

Prochaska JJ, Das S, Young-Wolff KC: Smoking, mental illness, and public health. Annu Rev Public Health 38:165–185, 2017 27992725

Ratschen E, Britton J, Doody GA, et al: Tobacco dependence, treatment and smoke-free policies: a survey of mental health professionals' knowledge and attitudes. Gen Hosp Psychiatry 31(6):576–582, 2009 19892217

Scanlon PD, Connett JE, Waller LA, et al: Smoking cessation and lung function in mild-to-moderate chronic obstructive pulmonary disease. Am J Respir Crit Care Med 161(2 Pt 1):381–390, 2000 10673175

Slade J, Bero LA, Hanauer P, et al: Nicotine and addiction: the Brown and Williamson documents. JAMA 274(3):225–233, 1995 7609231

Smith PH, Mazure CM, McKee SA: Smoking and mental illness in the U.S. population. Tob Control 23(e2):e147–e153, 2014 24727731

Sparrock LS, Phan L, Chen-Sankey J, et al: Nicotine pouch: awareness, beliefs, use, and susceptibility among current tobacco users in the United States, 2021. Int J Environ Res Public Health 20(3):2050, 2023 36767414

Sun R, Mendez D, Warner KE: Trends in nicotine product use among US adolescents, 1999–2020. JAMA Netw Open 4(8):e2118788, 2021 34432013

Thun MJ, Apicella LF, Henley SJ: Smoking vs other risk factors as the cause of smoking-attributable deaths: confounding in the courtroom. JAMA 284(6):706–712, 2000 10927778

United States Public Health Service Office of the Surgeon General, National Center for Chronic Disease Prevention and Health Promotion (US) Office on Smoking and Health: Smoking Cessation: A Report of the Surgeon General. Washington, DC, U.S. Department of Health and Human Services, 2020. Available at: https://www.ncbi.nlm.nih.gov/books/NBK555591. Accessed August 4, 2024.

Wang TW, Asman K, Gentzke AS, et al: Tobacco product use among adults—United States, 2017. MMWR Morb Mortal Wkly Rep 67(44):1225–1232, 2018 30408019

White JL, Conner BT, Perfetti TA, et al: Effect of pyrolysis temperature on the mutagenicity of tobacco smoke condensate. Food Chem Toxicol 39(5):499–505, 2001 11313117

World Health Organization: Tobacco or Health: A Global Status Report. Geneva, World Health Organization, 1997

Yuan S, Titova OE, Damrauer SM, et al: Swedish snuff (snus) dipping, cigarette smoking, and risk of peripheral artery disease: a prospective cohort study. Sci Rep 12(1):12139, 2022 35840660

2

Non-Cigarette Tobacco Products

Health Risks, Addictiveness, and Patterns of Use

At the end of the twentieth century, more than 90% of the worldwide sales of tobacco products consisted of cigarettes (including manufactured and roll-your-own cigarettes), amounting to more than 5 trillion cigarettes per year (Asma et al. 2014). In 2000, approximately 88% of tobacco sales in the United States were cigarettes, 2% were cigars, and 10% was smokeless tobacco, largely consisting of moist snuff products (Nkosi et al. 2022). At that time, most efforts by both clinicians and tobacco control public health professionals were focused on helping people who smoked cigarettes to quit and on trying to reduce the uptake of smoking among young people. The evidence at that time suggested that many people who smoked cigars "primarily" smoked cigarettes and inhaled cigar smoke as they did cigarette smoke, thus sustaining comparable health effects. Although less scientific evidence was available about the health effects of moist snuff, each can of snuff carried warnings about oral cancer, so it was widely believed to be about as harmful as cigarettes. However, by the beginning of the twenty-first century, the tobacco industry had begun to develop a much wider range of products, and evidence began to emerge of meaningful differences in both the harms to health and the addictiveness of these products. The tobacco industry—which at that time was primarily the cigarette industry—had begun to lose product liability lawsuits, and the publicity and effects of those losses resulted in reductions in cigarette smoking. In the United States, two of the biggest effects resulted from 1) the Master Settlement Agreement (MSA) and 2) the Engle class-action lawsuit based in Florida.

The MSA was finalized in November 1998 following negotiations between the attorneys general of 46 U.S. states and the four largest cigarette manufacturers. The states had sued the tobacco companies for recovery of their tobacco-related Medicaid costs (state-based health insurance). The settlement was complex but required these companies to continue to compensate each state in approximate proportion to their respective cigarette sales moving forward. By 2022, the states had received more than $150 billion, and these payments will continue annually for as long as the companies continue selling cigarettes (Jayawardhana et al. 2014). Another part of the MSA was the establishment of a national public health foundation dedicated to preventing youth tobacco use and helping people's efforts to quit. This was initially called the American Health Foundation and was later renamed the Truth Initiative after a highly effective national antismoking media campaign (Graham 2020).

The Engle class action lawsuit initially resulted in a $145 billion verdict for the plaintiffs (a large number of Floridians addicted to smoking) in May 2003, and although it was partially overturned on appeal (requiring individual plaintiffs to prove their cases) (Cummings et al. 2006), these two large defeats for the tobacco industry (MSA and Engle) forced it to raise the price of cigarettes (reducing consumption) and to more seriously look for other, potentially less harmful (and less costly) ways to stay in business.

Another key development that influenced the availability of alternative tobacco products in the United States was the signing of the Family Smoking Prevention and Tobacco Control Act in June 2009. This Act authorized the FDA to regulate the content, marketing, and sale of tobacco products. It banned the use of expressions such as "light" or "mild" to describe cigarettes in a way that falsely gave the impression of being less harmful. However, the Act also created a legal framework for tobacco companies to create reduced-harm products and to apply to the FDA for the right to claim that the product was a "modified-risk tobacco product" (MRTP) (Zeller 2012).

In parallel with these developments, nicotine/tobacco products have become more diverse, moving beyond cigarettes, and over time the FDA has obtained the legal authority to regulate these products. As shown in Chapter 1, the uptake of cigarette smoking by teenagers has declined markedly since 1997 but has been partially replaced by the use of non-cigarette tobacco products. This suggests that in the coming years, nicotine use among young people will mainly be via such products (e.g., electronic [e-]cigarettes). In this chapter, we describe each of these products before discussing the clinical implications for assessing and treating the patients who use them.

Electronic Cigarettes

An e-cigarette (also known as an e-cig, vape, vape pen, electronic nicotine delivery system, and other names) is a small, battery-powered device containing a heating element (coil) that heats a liquid solution containing nicotine to produce an aerosol that can be inhaled via a mouthpiece. The liquid typically comprises propylene glycol or glycerin plus nicotine as well as flavoring. The e-cigarette aerosol typically contains far fewer numbers and lower levels of toxicants than cigarette smoke (Hartmann-Boyce et al. 2023; McNeill et al. 2022), and for this reason, they appear to pose far lower health risks than combustible cigarettes (McNeill et al. 2022; Rigotti 2018). E-cigarettes only became widely available on the U.S. market around 2010 and have changed rapidly since then (Regan et al. 2013). Their long-term health effects are therefore unknown and must be estimated based on current and ongoing research evidence.

In 2020, e-cigarettes were the second most commonly used nicotine/tobacco product, with 3.7% of adults using them "every day" or "some days." The vast majority of adult users were current or former cigarette users, and more than 75% stated that their reason for using e-cigarettes was to either reduce or quit their cigarette smoking (Wackowski et al. 2016). The evidence from both randomized controlled trials (Hartmann-Boyce et al. 2023) and population research suggests that regular e-cigarette use can help people quit smoking (Warner et al. 2023). Of particular public health relevance, the evidence suggests that use of e-cigarettes (particularly those with nicotine delivery close to that of a cigarette) among people who smoke daily and have no plans to quit results in an increased probability of subsequent smoking cessation (Foulds et al. 2022; Kasza et al. 2021).

Concerns about e-cigarettes peaked in 2019, when their monthly use by teenagers was as high as approximately 25%. That year, there was also an outbreak of serious lung diseases in the United States that were initially suspected of being caused by the use of e-cigarettes and were therefore called "e-cigarette or vaping use–associated lung injury," or EVALI. However, it soon became clear that this lung disease was caused by vitamin E acetate being added to illicit Δ^9-tetrahydro-cannabinol (Δ^9-THC) vapes and not by nicotine e-cigarette use (Hall et al. 2021). Although numerous THC vapes used by people with EVALI were found to contain vitamin E acetate, no nicotine e-cigarette was ever found to contain it, and the number of cases of EVALI reduced rapidly by the end of 2019 despite nicotine e-cigarettes continuing to be widely used (Blount et al. 2020). The EVALI outbreak and the ongoing confusion about its causes underline the importance of clarifying the nature of the substance and the type of vaping device being used (e.g., THC vape or nicotine e-cigarette) when assessing vaping in patients.

The types of e-cigarettes being used, particularly by young people, have changed rapidly since they first became available. From 2010 to 2014, most people first tried using "cigalike" e-cigarettes that resembled a cigarette in appearance but were subsequently shown to deliver relatively low levels of nicotine (Yingst et al. 2019a). During that time, more experienced users learned that larger devices with more powerful batteries (sometimes referred to as "box mods") were more effective in delivering nicotine (Wagener et al. 2017), as were some types of vape pens (Hiler et al. 2017). In 2015, a new type of e-cigarette called Juul was launched that revolutionized the market. The Juul is a small e-cigarette about the size of a computer flash drive that contains a higher concentration of nicotine in salt form. The Juul also includes circuitry that controls the temperature of the heating element. The combination of its size, ease of use (breath activated), and high nicotine delivery (Yingst et al. 2019b) make the Juul very popular, particularly among young people, and this has sparked a range of similarly designed imitators, sometimes referred to as "pod mods" or "salt-nicotine pod devices" because the nicotine salt is typically contained in a disposable pod rather than a cartridge (Lee et al. 2020). In 2019–2020, disposable salt-nicotine devices containing various flavors became popular after Juul stopped selling flavors other than tobacco and menthol flavor (Figure 2–1).

The FDA required all e-cigarette manufacturers to apply for permission to stay on the market by September 2020. They received more than 6 million applications (e.g., for devices, liquids, flavors, cartridges), and by July 2024, more than 98% of these had been denied. Only a handful of

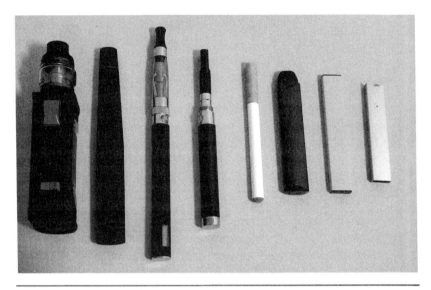

Figure 2–1. Examples of the range of different styles and designs of electronic cigarettes.

devices were authorized to remain on the market. No flavored e-cigarette liquids other than tobacco or menthol flavor had been approved as of July 2024. Less than 2% of the original e-cigarette marketing applications were still undecided by that time, and these products have been allowed to remain on the market until a final decision is made.

Given that e-cigarettes remain easily accessible and widely used and that the FDA has now authorized multiple e-cigarette brands to be marketed, implying that their availability is "appropriate for the protection of public health," it appears likely that they will continue to be widely used for the foreseeable future in the United States and around the world. While these products remain controversial, growing consensus suggests that—although they are not harmless and should not be used by people who do not smoke—they are significantly less harmful than combustible tobacco products and can help people quit smoking (Hartmann-Boyce et al. 2022; McNeill et al. 2022).

Cigars

Cigars are different from cigarettes in that, rather than the tobacco being wrapped in paper, it is wrapped in a material that includes

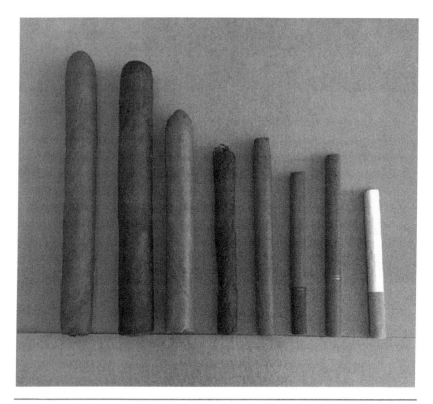

Figure 2–2. Examples of different sizes and types of cigars (e.g., filtered vs. non-filtered) compared with a typical cigarette (*right*).
Source. National Academies of Sciences, Engineering, and Medicine: Premium Cigars: Patterns of Use, Marketing, and Health Effects. Washington, DC, National Academies Press, 2022. Used with permission (CCC).

tobacco leaf (Figure 2–2). Cigars are traditionally (but not necessarily) larger than cigarettes and include various types, such as filtered cigars, little cigars, cigarillos, and large/traditional cigars. Like cigarettes, cigars are lit, and the smoke is often inhaled, so they potentially have similar health risks to cigarettes (Reilly et al. 2018). Conclusive evidence shows that the toxicants and carcinogens in cigar smoke, in general, are qualitatively the same as those in cigarette smoke.

In 2020, 3.5% of U.S. adults smoked cigars "every day or some days," with a sizable difference between sexes: 6.3% of men versus 0.8% of women (Cornelius et al. 2022). Since the late 1990s, overall cigar consumption has increased every year, with a total increase of 145%

between 1998 and 2020. Overall, evidence suggests that cigars are likely to be equally as harmful and addictive as cigarettes.

Smokeless Tobacco

The use of smokeless tobacco of various varieties is common throughout the world, with chewing tobacco and snuff being commonly used in North America, snus (a form of moist snuff that is low in nitrosamines and other toxicants) common in Sweden, and paan and gutka common in Southeast Asia. All of the commonly used varieties deliver pharmacologically active doses of nicotine, primarily via the lining of the mouth (with nasal snuff sometimes used in Europe). These different types vary as much as 130-fold in their content and delivery of tobacco toxicants (McNeill et al. 2006). Some (primarily Asian varieties) have very high concentrations of nitrosamines and are therefore a significant cause of oral cancer (Stepanov et al. 2005), whereas others, including the Swedish snus, have relatively low concentrations of nitrosamines and appear not to cause oral cancer (Foulds and Kozlowski 2007).

Given the harmful effects of nicotine on the fetus, all of these nicotine/tobacco products are potentially harmful in pregnancy. It has been proposed that the low-nitrosamine snus is around 90% less harmful to health than smoking (Levy et al. 2006) and has had a net beneficial effect on the health of Swedish men by helping reduce the number of people who smoke daily (Foulds et al. 2003). The significantly less harmful effects of snus compared with cigarettes were recently accepted by the FDA, when eight varieties of the Swedish Match brand General Snus were authorized as MRTPs in 2019 (Wackowski et al. 2021). This product is now authorized to include the following statement in its marketing: "No tobacco product is safe, but this product presents substantially lower risks to health than cigarettes."

Despite the MRTP authorization, presently there is little indication that the smokeless tobacco category is growing more than gradually, and there remains a large sex difference in use (4.5% of men and 0.3% of women in 2020). The one exception is the recent development of the "tobacco-free nicotine pouch" smokeless tobacco category. Nicotine pouches are prefilled microfiber pouches containing nicotine powder that dissolves in the mouth without requiring spitting (Sparrock et al. 2023). They do not contain tobacco but still fall under the regulatory authority of the FDA's Center for Tobacco Products because they contain nicotine and make no therapeutic claims. Their "tobacco-free" claims and white pouch coloring may make them more appealing to women than the otherwise similar portion–packed smokeless tobacco. Nicotine pouches entered the U.S. national market recently, and unit sales (a unit is one container with 15–20 pouches) increased from 163,000 in 2016 to 46 million in the first 6 months of 2020, with the Swedish Match product Zyn being the clear market leader, and mint/wintergreen flavors being the most popular. In early 2021, nicotine pouches were described as one of the fastest-growing tobacco product categories, with 5.6% of people who smoke having already tried them and 17% reporting interest in using them within the next 6 months. To date, neither the U.S. public nor tobacco researchers have a clear understanding of the risks and benefits of nicotine pouches to public health (Hrywna et al. 2022).

Pipes

Pipe smoking has been on a fairly consistent and gradual decline over recent decades, and pipes were used "every day or some days" by only 1.1% of the U.S. adult population in 2020 (1.5% of men and 0.7% of women) (Cornelius et al. 2022). Pipe smoking carries significant health risks similar to those of cigar smoking. Compared with no tobacco use, pipe smoking is associated with increased risk for cancer (oral, esophageal, larynx, and lung), coronary heart disease, stroke, and chronic obstructive pulmonary disease (COPD) (Henley et al. 2004; Shaper et al. 2003). Like other smoked tobacco products, the risk increases with the depth of inhalation and level of consumption (i.e., number of pipes smoked and years of smoking). Pipe smoke is more alkaline than cigarette smoke and dissolves more easily in saliva, thus reducing inhalation. Therefore, pipes deliver nicotine without the need to inhale and are capable of providing levels high enough to produce addiction and dependence. People who smoke pipes who formerly smoked cigarettes and continue their cigarette inhalation behaviors with pipes are at greater risk for tobacco-caused disease than those who primarily smoke pipes and have never smoked cigarettes (Ockene et al. 1987).

Heat-Not-Burn Cigarettes

A non-combusted "heat-not-burn" cigarette consists of a heating source and tobacco. The tobacco may be wrapped in paper, which makes it a type of cigarette. However, it is heated to a lower temperature than a combusted cigarette to create an aerosol that the user inhales, without any smoke (Bitzer et al. 2020). One such product, IQOS, was marketed in the United States in 2020 and was authorized as an MRTP by the FDA on the basis that it heats the tobacco without burning it and thus significantly reduces the production of harmful and potentially harmful chemicals. Because of a patent dispute with another tobacco company, IQOS was temporarily withdrawn from the U.S. market, but it and other brands of heat-not-burn cigarettes are still being sold in many other parts of the world and have gained a significant market share in some countries (e.g., Japan) (Odani and Tabuchi 2022), so it appears likely that they will reappear in the United States.

Because each of the products we have described in this chapter delivers nicotine, they all have the potential to be addictive. However, very few of them fully match the speed and concentration of nicotine delivery of a cigarette, so many are likely to be at least slightly less addictive (Figure 2–3). Because it typically requires decades of tobacco use for the full health effects of use to manifest (e.g., COPD, lung cancer), the overall health effects of tobacco products are a result of both the addictiveness and the toxicity of the product. Many of these alternative tobacco products have been developed only recently, and they all have significantly less research evidence into their harms and addictiveness than cigarettes. As a result, tobacco researchers have sometimes attempted to estimate their net harmfulness (Nutt et al. 2014). There is a broad consensus that combusted tobacco products are likely far more harmful to health than non-combusted nicotine/tobacco products (Centers for Disease Control and Prevention et al. 2010) and that the magnitude of the risk differences can be large. For example, a recent comprehensive review of the effects of e-cigarettes concluded that regular cigarettes are likely about 20 times more harmful than e-cigarettes (McNeill et al. 2022).

Case Example

Fiona (age 27) attended her first annual checkup with her family doctor in years because she and her husband had decided it was time to start a family, and she wanted to be as healthy as possible. She was glad that she had never picked up cigarette smoking because both of her parents had picked it up in their teens and were still smoking. When asked if she used any drugs, she replied, "No, a few glasses of wine when socializing on the weekend," and that she vaped, but only nicotine e-cigarettes, never anything with THC or other drugs. Although it is true that nicotine e-cigarettes are likely far less harmful than smoking,

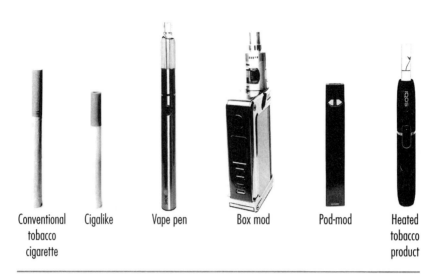

| Conventional tobacco cigarette | Cigalike | Vape pen | Box mod | Pod-mod | Heated tobacco product |

Figure 2–3.   Typical electronic nicotine delivery system (ENDS) devices showing different generations of electronic cigarettes and IQOS, a heated tobacco product.

Source.   Benowitz NL, St Helen G, Liakoni E: "Clinical Pharmacology of Electronic Nicotine Delivery Systems (ENDS): Implications for Benefits and Risks in the Promotion of the Combusted Tobacco Endgame." *Journal of Clinical Pharmacology* 61(Suppl 2):S18–S36, 2021. Used with permission (CCC).

including during pregnancy, nicotine itself can affect the development of the unborn child and should be avoided.

What Are the Concerns in This Case?

Many users of non-smoked nicotine products may correctly believe that their use of oral nicotine products or e-cigarettes is less harmful than smoking, but they may not be aware of the smaller but still potentially clinically meaningful additional risks from nicotine in specific clinical scenarios (e.g., pregnancy, recent stroke or myocardial infarction). In this case, Fiona should be informed that nicotine from e-cigarettes could be harmful to her baby during pregnancy and be offered assessment and treatment for potential nicotine dependence. The fact that she never smoked tobacco is important because it makes it extremely unlikely that she might initiate smoking while trying to quit vaping.

Key Points

- The pattern of use of nicotine products has changed significantly in the twenty-first century compared with the latter half of the twentieth century, in which cigarette smoking dominated.
- Although it is not easy to compare all potential long-term harms of traditional and novel nicotine products with precision, widespread consensus agrees that smoked products (particularly cigarettes) are likely significantly more harmful than non-smoked nicotine products.
- In the United States, the FDA can assess whether new nicotine products are appropriate for the protection of public health (and can be authorized for sale) and allow those products with sufficient scientific evidence to make claims that they present lower risk than traditional cigarettes.
- Use of non-cigarette and non-smoked nicotine products likely will continue to gain market share, and dual use of cigarettes and other products likely will continue to increase as more nicotine products are developed and as the scientific evidence on their risks and benefits develops.

References

Asma S, Song Y, Cohen J, et al: CDC Grand Rounds: global tobacco control. MMWR Morb Mortal Wkly Rep 63(13):277–280, 2014 24699763

Bitzer ZT, Goel R, Trushin N, et al: Free radical production and characterization of heat-not-burn cigarettes in comparison to conventional and electronic cigarettes. Chem Res Toxicol 33(7):1882–1887, 2020 32432464

Blount BC, Karwowski MP, Shields PG, et al: Vitamin E acetate in bronchoalveolar-lavage fluid associated with EVALI. N Engl J Med 382(8):697–705, 2020 31860793

Centers for Disease Control and Prevention, National Center for Chronic Disease Prevention and Health Promotion, Office on Smoking and Health: How Tobacco Smoke Causes Disease: The Biology and Behavioral Basis for Smoking-Attributable Disease. A Report of the Surgeon General. Atlanta, GA, Centers for Disease Control and Prevention, 2010

Cornelius ME, Loretan CG, Wang TW, et al: Tobacco product use among adults—United States, 2020. MMWR Morb Mortal Wkly Rep 71(11):397–405, 2022 35298455

Cummings KM, Brown A, Douglas CE: Consumer acceptable risk: how cigarette companies have responded to accusations that their products are defective. Tob Control 15(Suppl 4):iv84–iv89, 2006 17130628

Foulds J, Kozlowski L: Snus: what should the public-health response be? Lancet 369(9578):1976–1978, 2007 17498796

Foulds J, Ramstrom L, Burke M, et al: Effect of smokeless tobacco (snus) on smoking and public health in Sweden. Tob Control 12(4):349–359, 2003 14660766

Foulds J, Cobb CO, Yen M-S, et al: Effect of electronic nicotine delivery systems on cigarette abstinence in smokers with no plans to quit: exploratory analysis of a randomized placebo-controlled trial. Nicotine Tob Res 24(7):955–961, 2022 34850164

Graham AL: Engaging people in tobacco prevention and cessation: reflecting back over 20 years since the Master Settlement Agreement. Ann Behav Med 54(12), 932–941, 2020 33416838

Hall W, Gartner C, Bonevski B: Lessons from the public health responses to the US outbreak of vaping-related lung injury. Addiction 116(5):985–993, 2021 32364274

Hartmann-Boyce J, Lindson N, Butler AR, et al: Electronic cigarettes for smoking cessation. Cochrane Database Syst Rev 11(11):CD010216, 2022 36384212

Hartmann-Boyce J, Butler AR, Theodoulou A, et al: Biomarkers of potential harm in people switching from smoking tobacco to exclusive e-cigarette use, dual use or abstinence: secondary analysis of Cochrane systematic review of trials of e-cigarettes for smoking cessation. Addiction 118(3):539–545, 2023 36208090

Henley SJ, Thun MJ, Chao A, et al: Association between exclusive pipe smoking and mortality from cancer and other diseases. J Natl Cancer Inst 96(11):853–861, 2004 15173269

Hiler M, Breland A, Spindle T, et al: Electronic cigarette user plasma nicotine concentration, puff topography, heart rate, and subjective effects: influence of liquid nicotine concentration and user experience. Exp Clin Psychopharmacol 25(5):380–392, 2017 29048187

Hrywna M, Gonsalves NJ, Delnevo CD, et al: Nicotine pouch product awareness, interest and ever use among US adults who smoke, 2021. Tob Control 32(6):782–785, 2022 35217596

Jayawardhana J, Bradford WD, Jones W, et al: Master Settlement Agreement (MSA) spending and tobacco control efforts. PLoS One 9(12):e114706, 2014 25506827

Kasza KA, Edwards KC, Kimmel HL, et al: Association of e-cigarette use with discontinuation of cigarette smoking among adult smokers who were initially never planning to quit. JAMA Netw Open 4(12):e2140880, 2021 34962556

Lee SJ, Rees VW, Yossefy N, et al: Youth and young adult use of pod-based electronic cigarettes from 2015 to 2019: a systematic review. JAMA Pediatr 174(7):714–720, 2020 32478809

Levy DT, Mumford EA, Cummings KM, et al: The potential impact of a low-nitrosamine smokeless tobacco product on cigarette smoking in the United States: estimates of a panel of experts. Addict Behav 31(7):1190–1200, 2006 16256276

McNeill A, Bedi R, Islam S, et al: Levels of toxins in oral tobacco products in the UK. Tob Control 15(1):64–67, 2006 16436408

McNeill A, Brose LS, Robson D, et al: Nicotine Vaping in England: An Evidence Update Including Health Risks and Perceptions. London, U.K. Office for Health Improvement and Disparities, 2022. Available at: https://www.gov.uk/government/publications/nicotine-vaping-in -england-2022-evidence-update. Accessed August 4, 2024.

Nkosi L, Odani S, Agaku IT: 20-Year trends in tobacco sales and self-reported tobacco use in the United States, 2000–2020. Prev Chronic Dis 19:E45, 2022 35900882

Nutt DJ, Phillips LD, Balfour D, et al: Estimating the harms of nicotine-containing products using the MCDA approach. Eur Addict Res 20(5):218–225, 2014 24714502

Ockene JK, Pechacek TF, Vogt T, et al: Does switching from cigarettes to pipes or cigars reduce tobacco smoke exposure? Am J Public Health 77(11):1412–1416, 1987 3499090

Odani S, Tabuchi T: Prevalence of heated tobacco product use in Japan: the 2020 JASTIS study. Tob Control 31(e1):e64–e65, 2022 33707176

Regan AK, Promoff G, Dube SR, et al: Electronic nicotine delivery systems: adult use and awareness of the "e-cigarette" in the USA. Tob Control 22(1):19–23, 2013 22034071

Reilly SM, Goel R, Bitzer Z, et al: Little cigars, filtered cigars, and their carbonyl delivery relative to cigarettes. Nicotine Tob Res 20(Suppl 1):S99–S106, 2018 30125018

Rigotti NA: Balancing the benefits and harms of e-cigarettes: a National Academies of Science, Engineering, and Medicine report. Ann Intern Med 168(9):666–667, 2018 29435573

Shaper AG, Wannamethee SG, Walker M: Pipe and cigar smoking and major cardiovascular events, cancer incidence and all-cause mortality in middle-aged British men. Int J Epidemiol 32(5):802–808, 2003 14559754

Sparrock LS, Phan L, Chen-Sankey J, et al: Nicotine pouch: awareness, beliefs, use, and susceptibility among current tobacco users in the United States, 2021. Int J Environ Res Public Health 20(3):2050, 2023 36767414

Stepanov I, Hecht SS, Ramakrishnan S, et al: Tobacco-specific nitrosamines in smokeless tobacco products marketed in India. Int J Cancer 116(1):16–19, 2005 15756678

Wackowski OA, Bover Manderski MT, Delnevo CD, et al: Smokers' early e-cigarette experiences, reasons for use, and use intentions. Tob Regul Sci 2(2):133–145, 2016 27042688

Wackowski OA, O'Connor RJ, Pearson JL: Smokers' exposure to perceived modified risk claims for e-cigarettes, snus, and smokeless tobacco in the United States. Nicotine Tob Res 23(3):605–608, 2021 32812028

Wagener TL, Floyd EL, Stepanov I, et al: Have combustible cigarettes met their match? The nicotine delivery profiles and harmful constituent exposures of second-generation and third-generation electronic cigarette users. Tob Control 26(e1):e23–e28, 2017 27729564

Warner KE, Benowitz NL, McNeill A, et al: Nicotine e-cigarettes as a tool for smoking cessation. Nat Med 29(3):520–524, 2023 36788367

Yingst JM, Foulds J, Veldheer S, et al: Nicotine absorption during electronic cigarette use among regular users. PLoS One 14(7):e0220300, 2019a 31344110

Yingst JM, Hrabovsky S, Hobkirk A, et al: Nicotine absorption profile among regular users of a pod-based electronic nicotine delivery system. JAMA Netw Open 2(11):e1915494, 2019b 31730180

Zeller M: Three years later: an assessment of the implementation of the Family Smoking Prevention and Tobacco Control Act. Tob Control 21(5):453–454, 2012 22859058

3

Tobacco Use Disorder, Dependence, and Addiction

The continued use of tobacco and nicotine products is not merely a habit but the result of an addiction to nicotine caused by changes in the brain. Smoking or inhaling a substance into the lungs is a very effective way to deliver a high dose rapidly to the brain, making the nicotine from cigarettes highly addictive. Cigarettes are often trivialized because they are a legal substance or considered "not a real drug," yet nicotine is well documented to activate the brain reward pathways and to cause the release of dopamine in the nucleus accumbens, similar to other addicting substances.

Addiction has been defined in many ways, with most definitions including the core concept of chronic compulsive use of a substance despite it causing harm or the person having a desire to stop using the substance. The American Psychological Association website defined *addiction* in 2022 as "a state of psychological or physical dependence (or both) on the use of alcohol or other drugs. The term is often used as an equivalent term for substance dependence." The U.S. National Institute on Drug Abuse (NIDA) website stated in 2022 that "Addiction is a chronic disease characterized by drug seeking and use that is compulsive, or difficult to control, despite adverse consequences." The NIDA also warned about the stigma attached to certain words. It encouraged the use of terms such as "person with a tobacco use disorder" or "person with a nicotine addiction" rather than the terms "addict" or "user" (National Institute on Drug Abuse 2022).

The *Merriam-Webster Online Dictionary* (www.merriam-webster .com) provides both a medical and a lay definition of *addiction* as follows:

1. A compulsive, chronic, physiological or psychological need for a habit-forming substance, behavior, or activity having harmful physical, psychological, or social effects and typically causing well-defined symptoms (such as anxiety, irritability, tremors, or nausea) upon withdrawal or abstinence
2. A strong inclination to do, use, or indulge in something repeatedly

Dependence is often used as a synonym for *addiction* and is listed as such in the *Merriam-Webster Online Dictionary*. DSM-IV (American Psychiatric Association 1994) included the diagnosis of *tobacco dependence* and, in fact, made no mention of addiction because it was believed that the word had acquired a pejorative or stigmatized meaning. DSM-5 (American Psychiatric Association 2013) abandoned the terms *substance abuse* and *substance dependence* and instead introduced common criteria for all substance use disorders, requiring the presence of at least 2 of 11 criteria during the past 12 months.

Tobacco Use Disorder

Tobacco use disorder (TUD) is the diagnostic category within DSM-5 that most closely maps onto modern definitions of tobacco dependence or nicotine addiction. The 11 diagnostic criteria for TUD are listed in Table 3–1, alongside the six corresponding criteria used in ICD-10 for tobacco dependence (World Health Organization 1993).

Many definitions of addiction, like DSM-5's definition for TUD, are drawn from common definitions for other addictive substances. However, these definitions do not fit quite as well with tobacco addiction because 1) tobacco products are legal and relatively inexpensive, unlike many other addictive substances, and so tend not to result in legal problems; and 2) neither acute tobacco nor acute nicotine use typically causes the marked impairment in judgment or cognitive abilities (or driving abilities) that result from the use of many other addictive substances (e.g., alcohol or sedatives). Because many of the most serious health effects from smoking cigarettes (e.g., chronic obstructive pulmonary disease or lung cancer) are not evident until someone has smoked for decades, younger people who

Table 3–1. Summary of diagnostic criteria for tobacco use disorder from DSM-5 and tobacco dependence from ICD-10

DSM-5	ICD-10
A problematic pattern of tobacco use leading to clinically significant impairment or distress. Endorsement of at least two criteria in the past 12 months:	A cluster of behavioral, cognitive, and physiological phenomena in which the use of tobacco takes on a much higher priority than other behaviors that once had a greater value. Endorsement of three or more criteria present at some time during the past 12 months:
1. Tobacco is often taken in larger amounts or over a longer period than intended	
2. Persistent desire or unsuccessful efforts to cut down or control tobacco use	Difficulty in controlling tobacco use
3. A great deal of time is spent in activities necessary to obtain or use tobacco	
4. Craving, or a strong desire or urge to use tobacco	A strong desire to consume tobacco
5. Recurrent tobacco use resulting in a failure to fulfill major role obligations at work, school, or home (e.g., interference with work)	
6. Continued tobacco use despite having persistent or recurrent social or interpersonal problems caused or exacerbated by the effects of tobacco (e.g., argument with others about tobacco use)	

Table 3–1. Summary of diagnostic criteria for tobacco use disorder from DSM-5 and tobacco dependence from ICD-10 (*continued*)

DSM-5	ICD-10
7. Important social, occupational, or recreational activities are given up or reduced because of substance use	Progressive neglect of alternative pleasures or interests because of tobacco use, increased amount of time necessary to obtain or take tobacco or to recover from its effects
8. Recurrent tobacco use in situations in which it is physically hazardous (e.g., smoking in bed)	
9. Tobacco use is continued despite knowledge of having a persistent or recurrent physical or psychological problem that is likely to have been caused or exacerbated by tobacco	Persistent tobacco use despite clear evidence of harmful consequences
10. Tolerance: need for markedly increased amounts of tobacco to achieve the desired effect or markedly diminished effect with continued use of the same amount of tobacco	Evidence of tolerance, where greater tobacco use is needed to achieve the same effects originally produced by lower doses
11. Withdrawal: abrupt cessation of or reduction in the use of tobacco or a closely related substance, such as nicotine, followed within 24 hours by a) an increase in four or more of the seven characteristic withdrawal symptoms (see "Nicotine Withdrawal" section; see also DSM-5-TR criteria for tobacco withdrawal); or b) the substance is taken to relieve or avoid withdrawal symptoms	A physiological withdrawal state when tobacco use has ceased or been reduced, demonstrated by withdrawal or use of the same (or closely related) substance to avoid withdrawal symptoms

Note. DSM-5 specifies the TUD severity rating based on the number of criteria endorsed: two or three (mild), four or five (moderate), and six or more (severe).
Source. Derived from DSM-5 tobacco use and tobacco withdrawal criteria (American Psychiatric Association 2022) and *ICD-10 Classification of Mental and Behavioural Disorders: Clinical Descriptions and Diagnostic Guidelines* (World Health Organization 1992).

smoke may not have experienced many direct harms from their tobacco use, although they may be well aware that continued smoking can cause these harms. With some of the newer nicotine products (e.g., electronic [e-]cigarettes or oral nicotine pouches), the magnitude of the harms to health caused by chronic use has yet to be characterized, although it seems unlikely that their long-term use will ultimately be harmless.

Thus, a case can be made for adapting the traditional definition of *addiction* to retain the core components of chronic compulsive use without requiring known or experienced harmful consequences. Here we prefer to use the following definition of *nicotine addiction* and to use it as a synonym for *nicotine dependence* and *tobacco use disorder*:

> Nicotine addiction is a chronic disease characterized by continued nicotine seeking and use that is compulsive or very difficult to control, even if the person seriously tries to stop using or believes that continued use may be harmful.

With this definition, nicotine addiction can be identified by its behavioral characteristics even if the person has not yet made a serious quit attempt or has not yet experienced a serious health problem caused by their nicotine or tobacco use.

Clinical Features of Nicotine Addiction

When someone first tries a nicotine product, the more unpleasant subjective effects are often prominent, including dizziness and nausea, because the person will have no acquired tolerance to these effects and will not have learned appropriate dosing schedules (D'Silva et al. 2018). However, with repeated use, some people find the dizziness produced by the first cigarette of the day to be pleasurable, and some may describe it as a "rush" or "high." More typically, the positive subjective effects are relatively subtle and may only be noticeable after a few hours of abstinence. These positive subjective effects include feeling mild stimulation and improved ability to mentally focus, a pleasant calmness, less stress, and less hunger (Shiffman and Terhorst 2017).

Although some of these perceived beneficial effects are likely mediated by reduction of nicotine withdrawal symptoms (described in the "Nicotine Withdrawal" section that follows), some (e.g., improved cognitive performance) are also a primary direct result of nicotine's stimulatory effect, as demonstrated by the results seen in nonsmoking individuals who are given nicotine injections (Foulds et al. 1994, 1996). Continued nicotine use quickly causes the development of tolerance to its unpleasant effects (e.g., nausea), development of brain adaptations leading to upregulation of nicotinic receptors, and the experiences of withdrawal symptoms with abstinence and more marked positive subjective withdrawal relief when nicotine is again consumed after a short period of abstinence (e.g., overnight) (Benowitz 2010). People who smoke come to associate these perceived beneficial effects with the behavioral and sensory aspects of nicotine administration (e.g., lighting up a cigarette or feeling the throat scratch as smoke or aerosol hits the back of the throat with each puff), as well as with the situations in which nicotine is habitually consumed (e.g., when driving the car, talking on the phone, walking the dog). Both these associations and the internal states that feel similar to withdrawal symptoms (e.g., feeling sad, stressed, fuzzy-headed) can become triggers for cravings as the person learns that smoking a cigarette makes them feel better. In practice, however, when people who smoke cigarettes are asked about the effects they obtain from smoking on a normal afternoon without any abstinence period between cigarettes, they typically report only very mild sensations of "pepping up," "satisfaction," or "calming," and those subjective effects are felt less if the person was wearing a nicotine patch during the day (Foulds et al. 1992). It therefore appears that most of the positive effects of smoking are experienced intermittently following short periods of abstinence (a few hours or more), and that the primary driver of nicotine addiction is avoidance of unpleasant nicotine withdrawal symptoms.

Nicotine Withdrawal

One of the key characteristics of nicotine addiction is the onset of a characteristic set of unpleasant symptoms within 24 hours of a regular nicotine user abruptly ceasing use or significantly reducing their consumption. DSM-5 lists seven symptoms that are characteristic of nicotine withdrawal, and an increase in at least four of these is required for the diagnosis of nicotine withdrawal:

1. Depressed mood
2. Insomnia
3. Irritability, frustration, or anger
4. Anxiety
5. Difficulty concentrating

6. Restlessness
7. Increased appetite or weight gain

Other associated features include a craving for nicotine, a desire for sweets, impaired performance on tasks requiring vigilance, and slowing on electroencephalogram. Tobacco withdrawal can produce clinically significant mood changes and functional impairment (American Psychiatric Association 2022).

Time Course

Cognitive performance becomes impaired within 60 minutes of the last cigarette consumed, and subjective mood states become measurably worse within the same time frame and continue to worsen throughout the remainder of the day (Hendricks et al. 2006; Parrott et al. 1996). These nicotine withdrawal symptoms are relieved by nicotine replacement within the first 24 hours of abstinence (Fagerström et al. 1993; Hurt et al. 1998). A study of the effects of 12 hours of tobacco abstinence in aircraft pilots found marked impairments in mood and decision-making and concluded that "Abrupt cessation of smoking may be detrimental to flight safety, and the smoking withdrawal syndrome may influence flying parameters" (Giannakoulas et al. 2003).

There are many everyday situations in which a relatively brief (i.e., hours) period of abstinence from smoking may induce clinically significant nicotine withdrawal symptoms for which it may be advantageous for someone to use nicotine replacement. For example, a person who smokes regularly and has been admitted to a psychiatric hospital for observation and treatment after reporting suicidal ideation may report feeling more aggressive and depressed because of severe nicotine cravings and may benefit from receiving nicotine replacement therapy. In the context of a more extended period of abstinence, nicotine withdrawal symptoms peak around 24–48 hours of abstinence and then gradually subside over the next 3–6 weeks, with most clinically significant effects typically subsiding after 3 weeks.

Figures 3–1 through 3–4 show mean ratings by treatment condition (placebo or varenicline) and weeks after target quit date (TQD) for depressed mood (Figure 3–1); irritability, frustration, or anger (Figure 3–2); anxiety (Figure 3–3); and restlessness (Figure 3–4) (Foulds et al. 2013). Significant differences are evident between varenicline and placebo at weeks 1–6 and week 11 post-TQD. These data come from the largest ever placebo-controlled analysis of the time course of nicotine

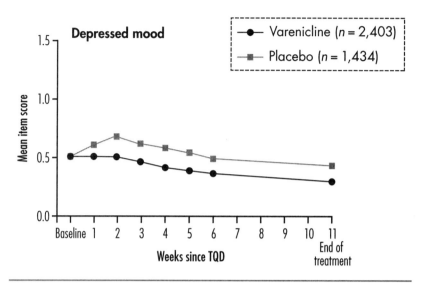

Figure 3–1. Time course of nicotine withdrawal symptoms over the first 11 weeks in people trying to quit smoking in double-blind, placebo-controlled trials of varenicline.

Mean ratings of depressed mood by treatment condition (placebo or varenicline) and number of weeks since target quit date (TQD). See Figures 3–2, 3–3, and 3–4 for additional data.

Source.   Foulds J, Russ C, Yu C-R, et al: "Effect of Varenicline on Individual Nicotine Withdrawal Symptoms: A Combined Analysis of Eight Randomized, Placebo-Controlled Trials." *Nicotine and Tobacco Research: Official Journal of the Society for Research on Nicotine and Tobacco* 15(11):1849–1857, 2013. Used with permission (CCC).

withdrawal symptoms in randomized double-blind trials ($N=3,837$) and include all patients attempting to quit smoking who attended their follow-up appointments, regardless of whether they had been completely abstinent from cigarettes during the prior week. Of the participants, 51% of the varenicline group and 23% of the placebo group were completely abstinent at week 6, but most had at least significantly reduced their cigarette consumption. Analyses focusing exclusively on participants with exhaled carbon monoxide levels consistent with abstinence tended to find that symptoms returned to baseline about 1 week earlier, but these likely excluded participants experiencing the most severe withdrawal symptoms. The ratings were made on a 0–4 scale in which 0=not at all, 1=slight, 2=moderate, 3=quite a bit, and 4=extreme. For each item, the increase from baseline was relatively

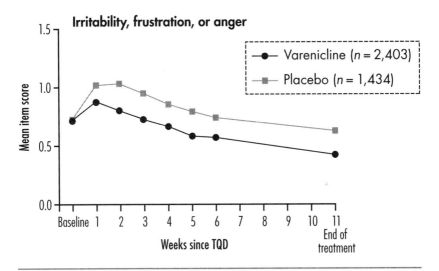

Figure 3–2. Time course of nicotine withdrawal symptoms over the first 11 weeks in people trying to quit smoking in double-blind, placebo-controlled trials of varenicline.

Mean ratings of irritability by treatment condition (placebo or varenicline) and number of weeks since target quit date (TQD). See Figures 3–1, 3–3, and 3–4 for additional data.

Source. Foulds J, Russ C, Yu C-R, et al: "Effect of Varenicline on Individual Nicotine Withdrawal Symptoms: A Combined Analysis of Eight Randomized, Placebo-Controlled Trials." *Nicotine and Tobacco Research: Official Journal of the Society for Research on Nicotine and Tobacco* 15(11):1849–1857, 2013. Used with permission (CCC).

small and equated to a rating of "slight." Of those in the placebo group who had item scores of 0–2 at baseline, the items rated as 4 (extreme) after they attempted to quit smoking were most commonly "urges to smoke" (7.4%) and irritability (6%). It appears that people are very sensitive to fairly small but perceptible changes in their mood and emotions and will take action to relieve even slight unpleasant symptoms, including resuming smoking during an attempt to quit.

Neurobiology of Tobacco Use Disorder/Nicotine Addiction

The psychological and behavioral effects of nicotine use are primarily the effects of nicotine from tobacco products on nicotinic acetylcholine

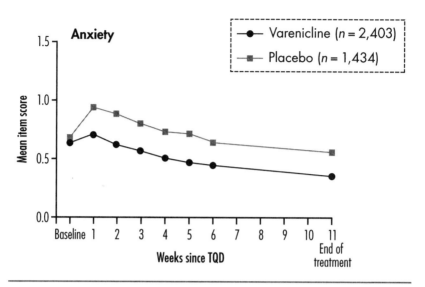

Figure 3–3. Time course of nicotine withdrawal symptoms over the first 11 weeks in people trying to quit smoking in double-blind, placebo-controlled trials of varenicline.

Mean ratings of anxiety by treatment condition (placebo or varenicline) and number of weeks since target quit date (TQD). See Figures 3–1, 3–2, and 3–4 for additional data.

Source. Foulds J, Russ C, Yu C-R, et al: "Effect of Varenicline on Individual Nicotine Withdrawal Symptoms: A Combined Analysis of Eight Randomized, Placebo-Controlled Trials." *Nicotine and Tobacco Research: Official Journal of the Society for Research on Nicotine and Tobacco* 15(11):1849–1857, 2013. Used with permission (CCC).

receptors (nAChRs) in certain parts of the brain. The subtype of nAChRs, composed of two α_4 and three β_2 subunits (Figure 3–5), is known to form the high-affinity binding sites in the brain (Foulds 2006). A particularly high concentration of α_4 subunits can be found in the ventral tegmental area (VTA) of the brain, where a dense supply of dopamine neurons is linked to the brain's main "reward center," the nucleus accumbens. When a sufficient concentration of nicotine is carried in the blood to activate $\alpha_4\beta_2$ receptors in the VTA, a burst firing of dopamine neurons occurs (Balfour 2004). The terminals of these neurons are in the medial shell and core areas of the nucleus accumbens. This stimulation of dopamine neurons causes an increased release of extrasynaptic dopamine in this area (Balfour 2004). The anatomical locations of these areas of the brain are shown in Figure 3–6.

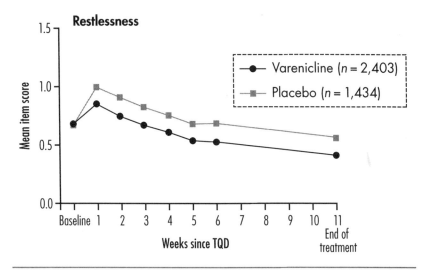

Figure 3–4. Time course of nicotine withdrawal symptoms over the first 11 weeks in people trying to quit smoking in double-blind, placebo-controlled trials of varenicline.

Mean ratings of restlessness by treatment condition (placebo or varenicline) and number of weeks since target quit date (TQD). See Figures 3–1, 3–2, and 3–3 for additional data.

Source. Foulds J, Russ C, Yu C-R, et al: "Effect of Varenicline on Individual Nicotine Withdrawal Symptoms: A Combined Analysis of Eight Randomized, Placebo-Controlled Trials." *Nicotine and Tobacco Research: Official Journal of the Society for Research on Nicotine and Tobacco* 15(11):1849–1857, 2013. Used with permission (CCC).

Repeated nicotine exposure results in an increase in functional nicotinic receptors in the brain and, specifically, a sensitization of the mesolimbic dopamine response to nicotine (Balfour 2004). This dopamine response (i.e., an increase in extrasynaptic dopamine in the extracellular space between fibers in the accumbens) appears to be associated with the reinforcing and addictive properties not only of nicotine but also of other psychostimulant substances of abuse (e.g., amphetamine, cocaine) (Pidoplichko et al. 1997). This response confers hedonic properties on the behaviors associated with dopamine activation. An animal that has experienced repeated nicotine boosts and accumbens dopamine stimulation by pressing a bar (or inhaling on a cigarette) will quickly learn that the behavior itself is enjoyable, and it comes to acquire reinforcing properties. Over time and repeated exposures, a

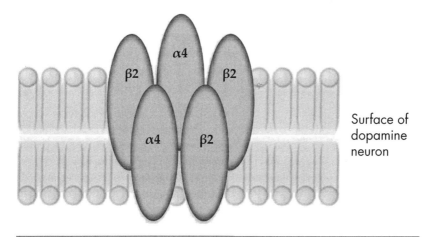

Figure 3–5. Simplified structure of an α_4 β_2 nicotinic receptor, located on the surface of a dopamine cell body.
Source. Foulds J: "The Neurobiological Basis for Partial Agonist Treatment of Nicotine Dependence: Varenicline." *International Journal of Clinical Practice* 60(5):571–576, 2006. Used with permission (CCC).

person's smoking ritual (e.g., opening the pack, lighting the cigarette, feeling the smoke hit the back of the throat) becomes capable of stimulating mesolimbic dopamine and therefore acts as a reinforcer itself, even in the absence of agonist (nicotine)-stimulated dopamine activation (Balfour 2004). This may be why people who smoke often state that they enjoy the "ritual" of smoking.

Salience refers to the state or quality to which something stands out from its neighbors. This is a key attentional mechanism that facilitates learning and survival by motivating the seeking of certain things. The D1 type spiny neurons in the shell of the nucleus accumbens are responsible for giving this motivational or incentive salience ("want" or "desire") to rewarding stimuli. After repeated use, the "liking" (pleasure or hedonic value) of a substance or other stimulus becomes dissociated from the "wanting" (i.e., desire or craving) due to the activation of incentive salience. As the incentive salience associated with consuming the substance becomes pathologically amplified, the person may begin to want the substance more and more while liking it less and less because tolerance quickly develops to its pleasurable effects. Behavior also shifts from being more impulsive to compulsive (George and Koob 2010). Early drug-seeking behaviors can then can be conceptualized as being motivated by positive reinforcement—or the desire to

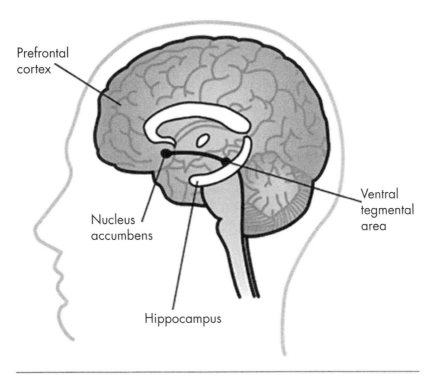

Prefrontal cortex

Nucleus accumbens

Ventral tegmental area

Hippocampus

Figure 3–6. Simplified diagram of the brain, showing the anatomic locations of the ventral tegmental area and the nucleus accumbens.

Source. Foulds J: "The Neurobiological Basis for Partial Agonist Treatment of Nicotine Dependence: Varenicline." *International Journal of Clinical Practice* 60(5):571–576, 2006. Used with permission (CCC).

feel pleasure or high—that is associated with activation of dopamine-mediated reward systems in the brain.

After repeated substance use, there is evidence of reduced dopamine activity in the reward pathways. This has been shown in brain imaging studies of not only nicotine users but also users of alcohol, cocaine, and methamphetamine (Koob 2013b). Addiction is paradoxically associated with lower dopamine concentrations and reduced reinforcement responses and can be considered a condition of brain reward deficit. This leads to reduced sensitivity not only to substances but also to natural rewards.

Alternate mechanisms have been proposed for the compulsive drug-seeking behavior that continues despite consequences from addiction and the likely reduced subjective experiences of pleasure. The term *negative reinforcement* refers to behaviors that seek to remove negative emotional states, uncomfortable or unpleasant feelings, or any type of subjective distress. The most frequent example of using substances to remove uncomfortable or unpleasant feelings is what happens when someone enters withdrawal. Because nicotine has a short half-life and leaves the body fairly quickly, a regular user can experience withdrawal within just 2–6 hours of their last use. The experience of physical withdrawal is a strong motivator to seek out and use substances, which continues the cycle of addiction through repeated intoxication and withdrawal. In addition to acute withdrawal, which may be intense and last for days to weeks, protracted abstinence may lead to persistent physiological, mood, and sleep changes that increase the risk for relapse.

Aside from withdrawal, other examples of negative reinforcement include using substances to overcome the effects of trauma or other mental illnesses, such as depression. Thinking about substance use at the societal level, patterns of use are consistently higher among populations with low socioeconomic status, suggesting that this is another form of negative reinforcement whereby individuals use substances to cope with the distress of poverty, discrimination, racism, or other neglect. An integrated model proposed by neuroscientist George Koob (2013a) represents the change in drug-seeking behavior (from positive to negative reinforcement) that occurs across the development of addiction (Figure 3–7).

At least three major brain areas are implicated in addiction. The rewarding structures of the mesolimbic dopamine pathways near the basal ganglia are only one part of a complex system that also includes the extended amygdala in the temporal lobe and the prefrontal cortex. Experiences of withdrawal, mood, and distress, termed *negative affect*, are localized in the extended amygdala, and withdrawal states are associated with activation of central adrenergic systems. Negative emotional states such as irritability, emotional pain, malaise, and dysphoria are directly related to relapse and contribute to using substances as a form of self-medication. The prefrontal cortex is responsible for complex functions including planning, decision-making, and understanding consequences. With repeated substance use, the functioning of the prefrontal cortex is disrupted and contributes to preoccupation with substance use and craving. Interactions in these three regions explain the repetitive cycle of substance use such as preoccupation/craving, binge/intoxication, and withdrawal (Koob 2013b).

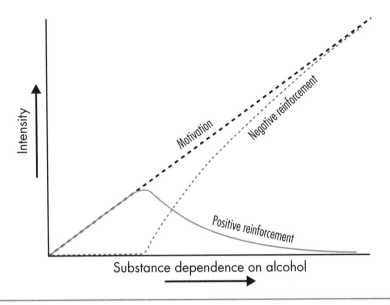

Figure 3–7. Theoretical framework relating addiction cycle to motivation for drug seeking.

This figure, from Koob 2013a, shows the change in the relative contribution of positive and negative reinforcement constructs during the development of substance dependence. This model originally used alcohol as the example drug, but it can be applied to nicotine and other dependence-forming drugs.

Source. Vendruscolo LF, Koob GF: "Alcohol Dependence Conceptualized as a Stress Disorder," in *Oxford Handbook of Stress and Mental Health*. Edited by Harkness K, Hayden EP. New York, Oxford University Press, 2019, pp. 1–37. Used with permission (CCC).

Changes in the frontal lobes may be particularly relevant to understanding the vulnerabilities and risks of substance use in young people. The brain has not completed the final processes of maturation, including pruning, until the age of 25, and because these processes occur from posterior to anterior, the frontal lobe is the last to mature. This suggests that many aspects of youth impulsivity, including seeking and using substances, are at least in part due to biological processes. The hedonic pleasure centers of the dopamine mesolimbic systems (located in the center of the brain) are mature before the inhibiting centers of the frontal lobe that weigh the consequences of substance use.

Figure 3–8 presents a greatly simplified model for a) nicotine activating nicotinic receptors and stimulating dopamine release; b) nicotine withdrawal decreasing dopamine release; and c) varenicline blocking nicotinic receptors, with the partial agonist effect producing moderate levels of dopamine release and reducing withdrawal and craving.

Clinical Implications of Nicotine Use as an Addictive Behavior

Surveys of adults and youth who smoke cigarettes typically find that more than 90% are aware that smoking can cause lung cancer and other serious illnesses. For this reason, at least 70% of people who currently smoke state that they would like to quit smoking, and around 40%–55% make a quit attempt lasting at least 24 hours each year. Unfortunately, only around 7% of those individuals in the United States report quitting each year (Walton et al. 2020), and people trying to quit smoking who participate in the placebo or control arm of randomized controlled trials of smoking cessation treatments typically have 1-year biochemically validated abstinence rates of 10% or less. One of the most thorough studies of population smoking cessation attempts across Australia, Canada, the United Kingdom, and the United States found that only 10% of adults who smoked had never tried to quit and that the average 40-year-old who started smoking in their teens will already have made more than 20 failed quit attempts. This speaks clearly to the difficulty of successfully quitting, even when most people who smoke have at some time abstained for at least 1 month before relapsing (Borland et al. 2012).

Although most people who smoke or have smoked in the United States successfully quit by the age of 60, the delays in smoking cessation mean that, each year, millions of newborn babies are affected by smoke exposure in utero, millions of adults experience smoking-caused diseases that could have been prevented by quitting earlier, and, of course, more than 400,000 die prematurely each year because of the cumulative effects of decades of smoking during their lifetime. A health professional simply advising patients that quitting smoking would improve their health, although much better than ignoring it completely, is unlikely to result in those patients being abstinent 1 year later. It is also clear that the reasons patients find it difficult to effectively follow such brief advice to quit is typically not that they have no desire or interest in quitting; the reality is that most want to quit and have tried unsuccessfully many times. The problem, which most people become aware of over time, is that they have become addicted

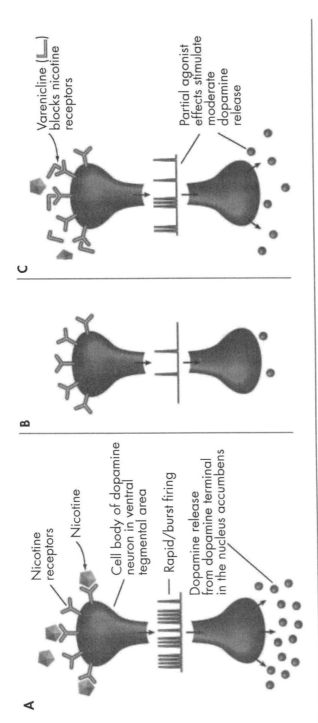

Figure 3–8. Greatly simplified model for a) nicotine activating nicotinic receptors and stimulating dopamine release; b) nicotine withdrawal decreasing dopamine release; and c) varenicline blocking nicotinic receptors, with the partial agonist effect producing moderate levels of dopamine release and reducing withdrawal and craving.

Source. Foulds J: "The Neurobiological Basis for Partial Agonist Treatment of Nicotine Dependence: Varenicline." *International Journal of Clinical Practice* 60(5):571–576, 2006. Used with permission (CCC).

to nicotine, and the challenge of overcoming that addiction may seem insurmountable. In the chapters that follow we describe how nicotine addiction can be assessed and how such assessment can be used to guide treatment.

Case Example

Jacob (age 35) works as an operating room nurse, often working 12-hour shifts and assisting with surgical procedures lasting many hours without a break. The hospital in which he works also prohibits any tobacco use within the grounds. Before he moved to the United States 10 years ago, he smoked a pack (20 cigarettes) a day, the first within 5 minutes of waking each day. Now Jacob typically smokes four cigarettes in the morning before starting work, with the last being smoked while he drinks a cup of coffee in a shop around the corner from the medical center immediately prior to starting his shift. He has noticed that, during the last few hours of these long shifts, he feels more stressed and irritable than he does in the morning. He believes this is caused by the stress and fatigue of his work. He typically lights up a cigarette as soon as he reaches his car at the end of his shift and smokes a few more during the drive home. Jacob and his wife have recently started a family, and he has agreed not to smoke in the home, so he now only smokes about 8–10 cigarettes per day.

What Are the Concerns in This Case?

Although Jacob currently smokes about 8–10 cigarettes per day, his past 20-per-day smoking history, his smoking as soon as he has the opportunity, and the likely onset of withdrawal symptoms toward the end of his shifts suggest that he is more addicted than his current consumption might suggest. Many people live and work in environments with tobacco use restrictions that limit their ability to smoke and may cause them to experience nicotine withdrawal symptoms on a daily basis. It can be helpful to explain to these patients that this can add stress to their lives and that it can be alleviated by quitting smoking with the help of a long-acting smoking cessation medication (discussed in later chapters, e.g., Chapter 7 and Chapter 10).

Key Points

- Nicotine dependence is characterized by the compulsive use of nicotine products.
- The other core characteristic of nicotine dependence is the onset of withdrawal symptoms when abstaining from all nicotine products.
- Nicotine withdrawal symptoms can onset within 6 hours of last use, peak within the first few days of abstinence, and typically return close to baseline within 3–4 weeks.
- Dependence lasts much longer than 1 month because former users are able to recall nicotine's reinforcing effects and are aware that their past use seemed to help with stress (when it was actually helping their nicotine withdrawal symptoms).
- Urges to use nicotine will recur long after the end of the acute nicotine withdrawal phase.

References

American Psychiatric Association: Diagnostic and Statistical Manual of Mental Disorders, 4th Edition. Washington, DC, American Psychiatric Association, 1994

American Psychiatric Association: Diagnostic and Statistical Manual of Mental Disorders, 5th Edition. Arlington, VA, American Psychiatric Association, 2013

American Psychiatric Association: Diagnostic and Statistical Manual of Mental Disorders, 5th Edition, Text Revision. Washington, DC, American Psychiatric Association, 2022

American Psychological Association: Substance use, abuse, and addiction, Psychology Topics. Washington, DC, American Psychological Association, 2022. Available at: https://www.apa.org/topics/substance -use-abuse-addiction. Accessed October 2024.

Balfour DJK: The neurobiology of tobacco dependence: a preclinical perspective on the role of the dopamine projections to the nucleus accumbens (corrected). Nicotine Tob Res 6(6):899–912, 2004 15801566

Benowitz NL: Nicotine addiction. N Engl J Med 362(24):2295–2303, 2010 20554984

Borland R, Partos TR, Yong H-H, et al: How much unsuccessful quitting activity is going on among adult smokers? Data from the International Tobacco Control Four Country cohort survey. Addiction 107(3):673–682, 2012 21992709

D'Silva J, Cohn AM, Johnson AL, et al: Differences in subjective experiences to first use of menthol and nonmenthol cigarettes in a national sample of young adult cigarette smokers. Nicotine Tob Res 20(9):1062–1068, 2018 29059351

Fagerström KO, Schneider NG, Lunell E: Effectiveness of nicotine patch and nicotine gum as individual versus combined treatments for tobacco withdrawal symptoms. Psychopharmacology (Berl) 111(3):271–277, 1993 7870963

Foulds J: The neurobiological basis for partial agonist treatment of nicotine dependence: varenicline. Int J Clin Pract 60(5):571–576, 2006 16700857

Foulds J, Stapleton J, Feyerabend C, et al: Effect of transdermal nicotine patches on cigarette smoking: a double blind crossover study. Psychopharmacology (Berl) 106(3):421–427, 1992 1570391

Foulds J, McSorley K, Sneddon J, et al: Effect of subcutaneous nicotine injections of EEG alpha frequency in non-smokers: a placebo-controlled pilot study. Psychopharmacology (Berl) 115(1–2):163–166, 1994 7862890

Foulds J, Stapleton J, Swettenham J, et al: Cognitive performance effects of subcutaneous nicotine in smokers and never-smokers. Psychopharmacology (Berl) 127(1):31–38, 1996 8880941

Foulds J, Russ C, Yu C-R, et al: Effect of varenicline on individual nicotine withdrawal symptoms: a combined analysis of eight randomized, placebo-controlled trials. Nicotine Tob Res 15(11):1849–1857, 2013 23694782

George O, Koob GF: Individual differences in prefrontal cortex function and the transition from drug use to drug dependence. Neurosci Biobehav Rev 35(2):232–247, 2010 20493211

Giannakoulas G, Katramados A, Melas N, et al: Acute effects of nicotine withdrawal syndrome in pilots during flight. Aviat Space Environ Med 74(3):247–251, 2003 12650272

Hendricks PS, Ditre JW, Drobes DJ, et al: The early time course of smoking withdrawal effects. Psychopharmacology (Berl) 187(3):385–396, 2006 16752139

Hurt RD, Offord KP, Croghan IT, et al: Temporal effects of nicotine nasal spray and gum on nicotine withdrawal symptoms. Psychopharmacology (Berl) 140(1):98–104, 1998 9862408

Koob GF: Addiction is a reward deficit and stress surfeit disorder. Front Psychiatry 4:72, 2013a 23914176

Koob GF: Theoretical frameworks and mechanistic aspects of alcohol addiction: alcohol addiction as a reward deficit disorder. Curr Top Behav Neurosci 13:3–30, 2013b 21744309

National Institute on Drug Abuse: Drug misuse and addiction, in Drugs, Brains, and Behavior: The Science of Addiction. Bethesda, MD, National Institute on Drug Abuse, 2022. Available at: https://nida.nih.gov/publications/drugs-brains-behavior-science-addiction/drug-misuse-addiction. Accessed September 2022.

Parrott A, Garnham NJ, Wesnes K, et al: Cigarette smoking and abstinence: comparative effects upon cognitive task performance and mood state over 24 hours. Psychopharmacology (Berl) 11(5):391–400, 1996

Pidoplichko VI, DeBiasi M, Williams JT, et al: Nicotine activates and desensitizes midbrain dopamine neurons. Nature 390(6658):401–404, 1997 9389479

Shiffman S, Terhorst L: Intermittent and daily smokers' subjective responses to smoking. Psychopharmacology (Berl) 234(19):2911–2917, 2017 28721480

Walton K, Wang TW, Prutzman Y, et al: characteristics and correlates of recent successful cessation among adult cigarette smokers, United States, 2018. Prev Chronic Dis 17:E154, 2020 33301394

World Health Organization: The ICD-10 Classification of Mental and Behavioural Disorders: Clinical Descriptions and Diagnostic Guidelines. Geneva, Switzerland, World Health Organization, 1992

World Health Organization: The ICD-10 Classification of Mental and Behavioural Disorders: Diagnostic Criteria for Research. Geneva, World Health Organization, 1993

4

Assessment of Tobacco Use and Tobacco Use Disorder

The optimal methods for assessing tobacco use depend to some extent on the context and reason for the assessment. Here we summarize some of the most widely used assessment methods in 1) research contexts (comprehensive assessments); 2) general medical contexts (e.g., family practice, general hospital intake); and 3) specialist substance use clinical services, including smoking cessation clinical services. We end by making recommendations for a brief core set of questions that should help identify clinically relevant tobacco/nicotine use, addiction, and interest in quitting or reducing consumption. The differences in methods used in these different contexts are partly driven by practical issues such as the time available to collect and analyze the information (higher in a research context) and the urgency of the need to quickly identify a feasible intervention that has a worthwhile chance of improving health outcomes (likely higher in a clinical context, in which the tobacco user may be presenting with a clinical problem caused by tobacco use and may be unusually responsive to the offer of treatment).

Comprehensive Tobacco Assessments in Research Contexts

When tobacco use is assessed in research contexts, whether it be national surveys of tobacco use behaviors or for eligibility of potential participants in clinical trials of tobacco treatment interventions, the process typically begins with some fairly standard screening questions designed to screen out nonusers. Research assessments typically use skip patterns in computerized assessments to avoid asking participants repeated questions about types of tobacco use that they have already indicated they have never used.

Tobacco/Nicotine Use and Products Used

In the United States, adult "never-users" are typically identified by asking, "Have you ever used a tobacco or nicotine product at least 100 times during your lifetime?" (e.g., National Health Interview Survey) (Holford et al. 2023). The assumption here is that if they have not used tobacco/nicotine at least 100 times in their life, they have not reached a level of frequency of tobacco/nicotine use likely to be clinically significant. Such individuals are typically excluded from further questions, unless the research is specifically aimed at understanding and preventing the uptake of problematic regular use (e.g., in studies of young people at ages before tobacco use has typically become established). To identify all of the tobacco/nicotine products that someone has ever used somewhat frequently, a question might include something like the following:

> Please check each of the following tobacco/nicotine products you have ever used at least 100 times in your life:
>
> ☐ Cigarettes (manufactured or "roll-your-own" cigarettes)
> ☐ Cigars (e.g., large cigar or little cigar/cigarillo)
> ☐ Smokeless tobacco (e.g., snuff, chew, or snus)
> ☐ Electronic cigarette (e.g., Juul, NJOY, nicotine vape, mod device)
> ☐ Hookah or waterpipe
> ☐ Pipe
> ☐ Heat-not-burn cigarettes (e.g., electronic product that heats tobacco without burning it, e.g., IQOS)
> ☐ Nicotine pouches (oral nicotine pouch product not containing tobacco, e.g., Zyn, On!, etc.)

- ☐ Nicotine replacement therapy products (e.g., nicotine patch, gum, lozenge, inhaler, spray)
- ☐ Traditional tobacco product (e.g., gutka or paan from Southeast Asia, Iqmik from Alaska)
- ☐ Other nicotine products (please list type of products you have used not mentioned above)

Subsequent questions then focus on products used recently:

> Please indicate which of these products you have ever used at least 100 times *and* have used either some days or every day during the past 3 months. (Person should indicate "No," "Yes, currently use every day," or "Yes, currently use some days.")

The period of time specified here may depend on the purpose of the project, ranging from the past 7 days to the past 12 months. Someone who last used a tobacco or nicotine product 3 weeks ago may commonly still be considered a "current user" based on the possibility that they may still be experiencing cravings to use or withdrawal symptoms and that there is a high likelihood of their continuing use. Past or former users can be identified as those who have ever used a specific product at least 100 times but who are not classified as current users because they are no longer using that product at all recently.

Frequency of Use

Common useful questions that can be asked to assess the frequency of use of every product currently being used include "On how many days out of the past 30 did you use [product]?" and "How many times per day do you typically use [product]?" Typically, this last question is best asked with a specific reference to both the time frame and the product itself. For example, "In the past 30 days, how many cigarettes have you smoked per day, on average?" For some products, the frequency of use may need to be defined, and this is often done in a manner designed to give a "cigarette equivalent." For example, for electronic (e-)cigarettes, the question might be, "How many times per day do you use an e-cigarette? (Assume one "time" lasts for around 10 minutes or consists of about 15 puffs)." The number of uses per day may not be easy to estimate; for most tobacco users, the number they provide should be used as a best estimate rather than as a precise measure. Even for cigarettes, people who smoke have a consistent tendency to exhibit "digit bias" by clumping their answers to 5, 10, or 20 per day, when their actual measured mean daily cigarette consumption (e.g., using ecological momentary assessment or returned cigarette butts) does not exhibit the same digit bias (Shiffman 2009).

Full Tobacco Use History

Depending on the purpose of the research project, a more detailed tobacco use history can be obtained by asking, for each product, about the 1) age when use started; 2) age when use ended; and 3) average daily consumption during the years of use. This level of information is not typically required outside research contexts, with the main exception being lung cancer screening, for which low-dose computed tomography (LDCT) imaging is recommended as an assessment for patients at high risk.

Tobacco Use Assessment in Medical Contexts

The U.S. Preventive Services Task Force recommends annual screening for lung cancer with LDCT for adults ages 50–80 years who have a 20 "pack-year" smoking history and currently smoke or who have quit during the previous 15 years. It is therefore common to estimate a patient's pack-year smoking history (i.e., number of cigarettes per day [CPD] multiplied by the number of years of smoking and then divided by 20) to identify whether they qualify for lung cancer screening. This estimation is typically a requirement before health insurance will pay for the screening (Liu et al. 2022). In practice, however, although a long pack-year history is a solid indicator of an increased risk for lung cancer (and therefore a likelihood to benefit from screening), it has very little value in determining how dependent the patient is or in providing much information relevant to helping them quit their smoking/tobacco use. Most general medical hospitals and family practices in countries such as the United States, Canada, and the United Kingdom conduct routine tobacco use screening at patient intake and annual checkups. Such screening information is often collected by administrative staff or the nurse responsible for collecting screening information before the patient is seen by their clinician. The screening questions are typically similar to those listed earlier (see "Comprehensive Tobacco Assessments in Research Contexts"), with slight variations in wording as periodically recommended and updated by The Joint Commission, the primary organization responsible for accrediting U.S. health care organizations and programs (Fiore and Adsit 2016).

Focus on Combustible Tobacco Products

Although no nicotine products are entirely free of risks (particularly during pregnancy), products that burn tobacco and produce smoke that users inhale (e.g., cigarettes, cigars, cigarillos, pipe tobacco, hookah) have the strongest evidence regarding their harms to health (see Chapter 1 and Chapter 2). Inhaling smoke exposes the user to a much larger spectrum of harmful chemicals and conveys a much greater risk to overall health than does the use of noncombustible tobacco products (e.g., snuff, chew, dip, nicotine pouches, e-cigarettes, heat-not-burn cigarettes). For this reason, in some clinical contexts, detailed assessment and intervention may sometimes focus on use of these more harmful products. However, all nicotine delivery products carry some risks, and these risks are typically a function of long-term regular use. For this reason, assessment of dependence or addiction to a specific tobacco or nicotine product is an important component of clinical evaluation.

Assessment of Dependence on Cigarettes

A number of questionnaire assessments of dependence on nicotine/tobacco use products have been developed. The most widely used questionnaire in smoking cessation research is the Fagerström Test for Cigarette Dependence (FTCD; sometimes called the Fagerström Test for Nicotine Dependence [FTND]) (Heatherton et al. 1991), a six-item questionnaire producing a score from 0 to 10 (Table 4–1).

Numerous studies have found that a baseline FTCD/FTND score is moderately predictive of which people are more likely to succeed in quitting smoking during an attempt (i.e., the lower the dependence score, the greater the chances of quitting). The score also has significant correlations with severity of withdrawal symptoms and biochemical measures of nicotine exposure (e.g., plasma cotinine) (DiFranza et al. 2012; Van Overmeire et al. 2016). Many studies have found that the two items on the FTND that measure the "Heaviness of Smoking Index" (CPD and time to first cigarette of the day) perform about as well as the total score from all six items in predicting quit success rates. This is shown in Figure 4–1 using pooled data from 2,763 people who smoked who were randomly assigned to varenicline and 2,229 who were randomly assigned to use placebo in 10 randomized,

Table 4–1. The Fagerström Test for Cigarette Dependence

Question	Answer	Score
How soon after you wake up do you smoke your first cigarette?	Within 5 minutes	3
	6–30 minutes	2
	31–60 minutes	1
	>60 minutes	0
Do you find it difficult to refrain from smoking in places where it is forbidden?	Yes	1
	No	0
Which cigarette would you hate to give up most?	The first one in the morning	1
	Others	0
How many cigarettes per day do you smoke?	≤10	0
	11–20	1
	21–30	2
	>30	3
Do you smoke more frequently during the first hours after waking than during the rest of the day?	Yes	1
	No	0
Do you smoke if you are so ill that you are in bed most of the day?	Yes	1
	No	0

Note. Scores are totaled to yield a single score. Typically 0–2 = very low, 3–4 = low, 5 = moderate, 6–7 = high, and 8–10 = very high dependence.
Source. Heatherton et al. 1991.

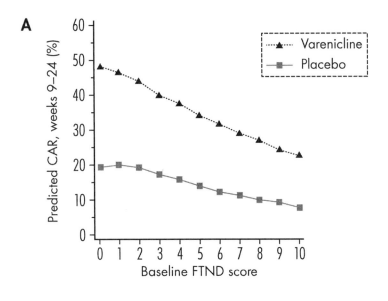

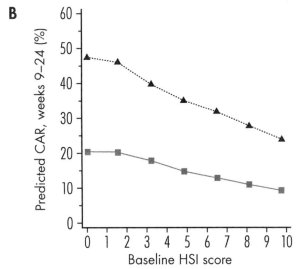

Figure 4–1. Predicted continuous abstinence rate (CAR) for weeks 9–24 by baseline (A) Fagerström Test for Nicotine Dependence (FTND) and (B) Heaviness of Smoking Index (HSI) scores.

Source. Fagerström K, Russ C, Yu C-R, et al: "The Fagerström Test for Nicotine Dependence as a Predictor of Smoking Abstinence: A Pooled Analysis of Varenicline Clinical Trial Data." *Nicotine & Tobacco Research: Official Journal of the Society for Research on Nicotine and Tobacco* 14(12):1467–1473, 2012. Used with permission (CCC).

double-blind, placebo-controlled trials of varenicline for smoking cessation (Fagerström et al. 2012).

The trials providing data for this analysis required a minimum smoking frequency of 10 CPD. However, these figures show that only around 20% of those treated with placebo, with an FTND score of zero at assessment, were continuously abstinent at 6-month follow-up. When 80% of those with the lowest possible score on the FTND are not able to quit, it suggests that the FTND may not be adequately measuring dependence at the lower end of the dependence continuum.

Relationship Between Frequency of Cigarette Consumption and DSM-5 Tobacco Use Disorder

Whereas DSM-IV (American Psychiatric Association 1994) required at least 3 of 7 criteria for the diagnosis of tobacco dependence, DSM-5 requires only 2 of 11 criteria to meet diagnostic criteria for tobacco use disorder (TUD) (American Psychiatric Association 2022). The 11 basic criteria for DSM-5, translated into an easy-to-administer questionnaire, are shown in Table 4–2. TUD is considered to be of "mild" severity when 2 or 3 criteria are met, "moderate" severity when 4 or 5 criteria are met, and "severe" when 6 or more criteria are met. One potential weakness of the FTND is that the questions bear little explicit relationship to DSM criteria for tobacco dependence (DSM-IV) or TUD (DSM-5) (Baker et al. 2012). However, a recent analysis of a representative sample of 6,793 people who smoked cigarettes exclusively found a close relationship between cigarette smoking frequency and severity of TUD (as assessed by the number of symptoms endorsed) (Oliver and Foulds 2021). As shown in Figure 4–2, even among those who smoked less than weekly, 18% of those who typically smoked only one or two cigarettes on a smoking day met TUD criteria. The figure shows a clear relationship between the frequency of cigarette smoking and the proportion of users who met DSM-5 TUD criteria, which becomes relatively flat above 10 CPD, at around 90%. Notably, almost two-thirds of those who smoked only one to four CPD met TUD criteria, as did most (64.1%) of those who smoked 3–6 days per week and a substantial minority (26.3%) of those who smoked less than once per week. DSM-5 states that TUD is considered to be of "moderate" severity when four or more criteria are met, and these data show this is typical at 10 CPD or more.

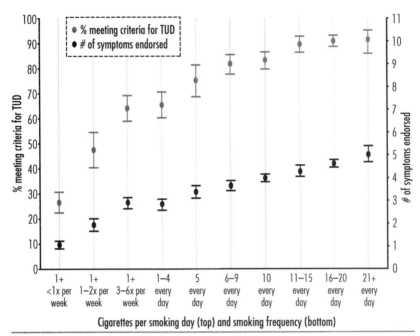

Figure 4–2. Relationship of cigarette smoking frequency with percentage of people who smoke meeting tobacco use disorder (TUD) criteria and the mean number of DSM-5 criteria/symptoms they met.

Source. Reprinted from Oliver JA, Foulds J: "Association Between Cigarette Smoking Frequency and Tobacco Use Disorder in U.S. Adults." *American Journal of Preventive Medicine* 60(5):726–728, 2021, with permission from Elsevier. Used with permission (CCC).

The results of this study highlight the high prevalence of TUD even among those whose smoking is considered to be "light" and the potential need for treatment within this population. Previous research has found that people who did not smoke daily were more likely than those who smoked daily to try to quit (Tindle and Shiffman 2011), but most of these attempts are not successful, even with nicotine replacement therapy (Shiffman et al. 2020). The overwhelming majority (85.0%) of people who smoke cigarettes daily and a sizable minority (44.0%) of those who smoke non-daily meet DSM-5 diagnostic criteria for TUD. Clinicians should ask patients about all smoking behaviors, including non-daily smoking, because even those who do not smoke daily may still require treatment to successfully quit smoking. Overall, research on the assessment of cigarette dependence suggests that clinicians can

---

Table 4–2. Questions that may be used to assess DSM-5 tobacco use disorder. There are 11 items, and each "yes" on items 1–10 counts as one criterion met, and at least four "yes" answers on item 11a OR a "yes" to 11b counts as one criterion met. Total score is number of criteria met out of 11.

The following questions are about experiences some people have had when using nicotine electronic (e-)cigarettes. Please answer "yes" to each question if this has happened to you in the past 12 months:

1. Did you have a period when you often used your e-cigarette more or longer than you intended to? Y N

2. Did you more than once TRY to stop or cut down on your e-cigarette use but found you couldn't do it? Y N

3. Did you have a time when you spent a lot of time making sure you had enough e-cigarette liquid/cartridges/pods/chargers available? Y N

4. Did you have a very strong desire or urge to use your e-cigarette? Y N

5. Did you continue to use your e-cigarette even though it was causing you problems at school or home or work? Y N

6. Did you continue to use your e-cigarette even though it was causing you problems in one or more relationships? Y N

7. Did you give up any activities that you were interested in or that gave you pleasure because e-cigarettes were not permitted at the activity or because you had spent required money on e-cigarettes instead? Y N

8. Did you more than once use an e-cigarette in a situation that could have been dangerous, for example, driving a car, riding a motorbike, using machinery, boating, etc.? Y N

9. Did you continue to use e-cigarettes even though you knew it was causing you a health problem or making a health problem worse? Y N

10. Did you increase your e-cigarette use because the amount you used didn't give you the same effect anymore? Y N

Table 4–2. Questions that may be used to assess DSM-5 tobacco use disorder. There are 11 items, and each "yes" on items 1–10 counts as one criterion met, and at least four "yes" answers on item 11a OR a "yes" to 11b counts as one criterion met. Total score is number of criteria met out of 11. (*continued*)

11a. When you cut down on heavy or prolonged use of e-cigarettes or stopped using for more than 24 hours, did you have any of the following withdrawal symptoms (four or more withdrawal symptoms required)?

Feeling irritable, frustrated, or angry	Y	N
Feeling tense or anxious	Y	N
Difficulty concentrating	Y	N
Increased appetite	Y	N
Feeling restless	Y	N
Feeling low or depressed	Y	N
Difficulty sleeping	Y	N
11b. Do you use e-cigarettes to reduce or avoid withdrawal symptoms?	Y	N

Source. Oliver and Foulds 2021.

adequately assess dependence by asking about patients' frequency of smoking and their time to their first cigarette of the day after waking. People who smoke 10 CPD or more or who smoke within 30 minutes of waking in the morning can be considered highly dependent. People who smoke 1–9 cigarettes daily but not within the first half-hour after waking can be considered moderately dependent, and those who smoke less often than daily (particularly <20 days over the past month) can be considered only mildly or nondependent. The greater the severity of dependence, the greater the likelihood that the patient will benefit from evidence-based treatment (counseling and pharmacotherapy).

Assessing Cigarette Dependence in Adolescents and Young Adults

The Hooked on Nicotine Checklist (Table 4–3) is a 10-item screening tool originally developed to assess loss of autonomy over tobacco in

Table 4–3. The Hooked on Nicotine Checklist

1. Have you ever tried to quit but couldn't?	○ Yes ○ No
2. Do you smoke now because it is really hard to quit?	○ Yes ○ No
3. Have you ever felt like you were addicted to tobacco?	○ Yes ○ No
4. Do you ever have strong cravings to smoke?	○ Yes ○ No
5. Have you ever felt like you really needed a cigarette?	○ Yes ○ No
6. Is it hard to keep from smoking in places where you are not supposed to (like school)?	○ Yes ○ No

When you tried to stop smoking or when you haven't used tobacco for a while…

7. Did you find it hard to concentrate because you couldn't smoke?	○ Yes ○ No
8. Did you feel more irritable because you couldn't smoke?	○ Yes ○ No
9. Did you feel a strong need or urge to smoke?	○ Yes ○ No
10. Did you feel nervous, restless, or anxious because you couldn't smoke?	○ Yes ○ No

The number of items checked "Yes" gives a total score, with 0 = no dependence, 1 = low dependence, and 10 = high dependence.

Source.   DiFranza et al. 2002.

adolescents who smoke and has become widely used to assess nicotine dependence in young people (DiFranza et al. 2002). Unlike the FTND, it does not require relatively heavy daily smoking (far less common in teenagers) to score, and it is designed to be sensitive to the early development of dependence by asking more questions about symptoms such as cravings and withdrawal symptoms. It consists of 10 Yes/No questions, with a score out of 10 for each "Yes" answer, which is interpreted as a "symptom" of dependence. The threshold for such answers is low, in that many of the questions ask if the person has "ever" experienced the symptom. This checklist has good psychometric properties, but most adults who smoke heavily tend to reach the ceiling score, so it is less sensitive at the high end of the dependence spectrum (Wellman et al. 2006).

Assessment of Dependence on Other Nicotine/Tobacco Products

Many of the assessments just described can be adapted to assess dependence on tobacco products other than cigarettes (Mushtaq and Beebe 2017). One assessment, the Penn State Nicotine Dependence Index (PSNDI), was specifically designed to use the most predictive items from the widely used cigarette dependence measures and to apply these in a questionnaire that could be used for other nicotine products by simply replacing the word *cigarette* with the product of interest. The PSNDI adapted the two items from the Heaviness of Smoking Index (Heatherton et al. 1989) to cover a wider spread of answers, particularly at the lower end of consumption (e.g., enabling scoring above zero for smoking ≤10 CPD, which is becoming much more common). The FTND was developed more than 20 years ago at a time when cigarettes were cheap and smoke-free workplaces were rare and, thus, daily cigarette consumption was higher. People whose cigarette consumption has been forced lower by these social changes may score low on the scale yet show other signs of dependence (e.g., repeated failed quit attempts). For example, the scoring scheme on the FTND for the cigarette consumption item (0–3) gives a zero score to anyone who smokes fewer than 11 CPD. Among people who smoke, Black individuals smoke an average of 10 CPD and Latiné people smoke an average of 7 CPD, yet they have low quit rates in clinical trials, suggesting that the current scoring scheme may be insensitive at lower levels of cigarette consumption, particularly for minority groups (Brook et al. 2009). In fact, 46% of Black people who smoke consume fewer than 10 CPD (vs. 19.3% of White people who smoke), but despite their lower cigarette consumption, they have significantly higher cotinine levels than White people who smoke (Caraballo et al. 2011). The Caraballo et al. (2011) study showed that, at lower levels of cigarette smoking (1–3 and 4–9 CPD), Black participants had serum cotinine levels almost 200% to 300% higher than that of White participants based on a representative population sample (from the National Health and Nutrition Examination Survey).

The cigarette version of the PSNDI was found to be at least as predictive of short-term cessation success as the FTND in a controlled trial of group treatment plus nicotine replacement (Foulds et al. 2015a), as shown in Figure 4–3.

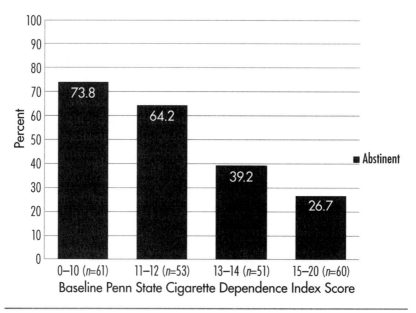

Figure 4–3. Percentage of people who smoke who were at least 7 days abstinent at 1-month follow-up (validated by exhaled carbon monoxide <10 ppm) by baseline Penn State Cigarette Dependence Index score.
Source.   Foulds et al. 2015a.

Scores on the e-cigarette version of this questionnaire (Foulds et al. 2015b), the Penn State Electronic Cigarette Dependence Index (PSECDI), were found to be correlated with the concentration of nicotine being used in the liquid in e-cigarettes and to predict which e-cigarette users had quit using them a year later (Piper et al. 2020; Sobieski et al. 2022), suggesting construct validity of the measure for e-cigarette users. Those allocated to a high-dose e-cigarette (36 mg/mL) in a double-blind randomized controlled trial had higher PSECDI scores after 6 months than those randomly assigned to zero or to 8 mg/mL, which also supports the validity of the questionnaire (Yingst et al. 2023). It also has shown good internal consistency (Pienkowski et al. 2022) and test-retest reliability after 1 month (+0.78) (Yingst et al. 2023) and correlates highly (around +0.7) with other measures of e-cigarette dependence (Morean et al. 2019). A study of 435 young (ages 18–30 years) e-cigarette users found that PSECDI score was highly predictive of still being a current user 12 months later, as shown in Figure 4–4 (Pokhrel et al. 2023).

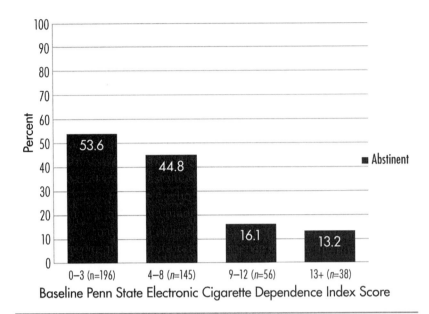

Figure 4–4. Percentage of young adult electronic cigarette users who self-reported that they no longer used electronic cigarettes in the past 30 days at 1-year follow-up, by baseline score on the Penn State Electronic Cigarette Dependence Index.
Source. Pokhrel et al. 2023.

The PSECDI questions are shown in Table 4–4. Items 1 and 2 are adapted from the Heaviness of Smoking Index items in the FTND. Items 3 and 4 are adapted from Bover et al. (2008), who found waking at night to use nicotine to be highly indicative of dependence. Items 5, 6, 8, 9, and 10 are adapted from the Hooked on Nicotine Checklist (DiFranza et al. 2002), and item 7 relating to strength of urges to use is adapted from Fidler and West (2011).

Biochemical Markers of Nicotine/ Tobacco Use and Dependence

Cotinine

Because nicotine in the blood/plasma peaks within minutes of nicotine product use and has a half-life of approximately 2 hours, a spot blood nicotine concentration is not particularly helpful in estimating

Table 4–4. Penn State Electronic Cigarette Dependence Index

1. How many times per day do you usually use your electronic cigarette (assume that one "time" consists of around 15 puffs or lasts around 10 minutes)?   _____ (Scoring: 0–4 times/day = 0, 5–9 = 1, 10–14 = 2, 15–19 = 3, 20–29 = 4, 30+ = 5)

2. On days that you can use your electronic cigarette freely, how soon after you wake up do you first use your electronic cigarette?   _____ (Scoring: < 5 minutes = 5, 6–15 = 4, 16–30 = 3, 31–60 = 2, 61–120 = 1, 121+ = 0)

3. Do you sometimes awaken at night to use your electronic cigarette?   _____ (Scoring: Yes = 1, No = 0)

4. If yes, how many nights per week do you typically awaken to use your electronic cigarette?   _____ (Scoring: 0–1 nights = 0, 2–3 nights = 1, 4+ nights = 2)

5. Do you use your electronic cigarette now because it is really hard to quit (using e-cigarettes)?   _____ (Scoring: Yes = 1, No = 0)

6. Do you ever have strong cravings to use your electronic cigarette?   _____ (Scoring: Yes = 1, No = 0)

7. Over the past week, how strong have the urges to use your electronic cigarette been?   _____ (Scoring: None/Slight = 0, Moderate/Strong= 1, Very Strong/Extremely Strong = 2)

8. Is it hard to keep from using your electronic cigarette in places where you are not supposed to?   _____ (Scoring: Yes = 1, No = 0)

When you haven't used an electronic cigarette for a while or when you tried to stop using…

9. Did you feel more irritable because you couldn't use your electronic cigarette?   _____ (Scoring: Yes = 1, No = 0)

10. Did you feel nervous, restless, or anxious because you couldn't use your electronic cigarette?   _____ (Scoring: Yes = 1, No = 0)

Table 4–4. Penn State Electronic Cigarette Dependence Index (*continued*)

11. What is the concentration of nicotine in the liquid that you usually use in your electronic cigarette?	_____ (Answers can be accepted in either percentage of nicotine or mg/mL. This does not contribute to the score but is often relevant to assessing dependence. Many e-cigarette users are unclear about the concentration.)

Source. Foulds et al. 2015b.
Note. Detailed instructions on use of the PSECDI can be found at: https://research .med.psu.edu/smoking/dependence-index.

total nicotine exposure. The result will depend on factors such as the time of day and the recency of last nicotine product use. On the other hand, the primary metabolite of nicotine, cotinine, has a half-life of around 16 hours and can be measured in various body fluids (blood, urine, saliva) (Benowitz et al. 2020). A spot saliva cotinine concentration greater than 10 ng/mL would indicate that the individual is highly likely (>95%) to have actively consumed a nicotine product in the past 2–5 days. The absolute cotinine concentration from a spot test can also provide a reasonable estimate of the amount of nicotine the person typically absorbs, which is related to their level of dependence. However, measurement of cotinine cannot identify the precise source of the nicotine (i.e., whether it was from a cigarette, smokeless tobacco, or nicotine replacement therapy). For this reason, cotinine and other nicotine metabolite measurements are mainly used in research studies, screenings for insurance policies (to confirm non–tobacco use status), and to verify nonsmoking status prior to certain types of surgery for which there is evidence of poor surgical outcomes among tobacco users.

Exhaled Carbon Monoxide

Burning organic matter gives rise to carbon monoxide as a byproduct of combustion. Carbon monoxide can be used as an indicator of recent smoke absorption from combustible tobacco products (e.g., cigarettes, cigars, pipes, hookah) but not smokeless tobacco or most electronic nicotine delivery systems. Its concentration can be measured in exhaled breath (exhaled carbon monoxide, or eCO) in parts per million (ppm) or in blood (carboxyhemoglobin in percent hemoglobin saturation). These two methods are very highly correlated (e.g., $r=0.95$) (Jarvis et al. 1986). eCO can be measured easily using a relatively inexpensive portable device, and this has become a widely used method for assessing tobacco smoke exposure and for validating self-reports of smoking cessation. Carbon monoxide levels must be assessed in the context of potential environmental exposures. In countries that largely ban smoking in public places and have relatively strong prohibitions on air pollution, people who do not smoke typically have an eCO in the lower part of the range, 0–5 ppm (Tual et al. 2010). However, in large industrial cities in countries without comprehensive smoke-free air policies, people who have never smoked often have eCO readings in the range of 2–8 ppm. Smoking marijuana is also a potential source because it produces carbon monoxide levels similar to tobacco smoking, and information on recent marijuana smoking should be elicited if possible when measuring participants' levels in research studies (Moolchan et al. 2005). Carbon monoxide typically has a half-life of around 4 hours, but this is influenced by pulmonary ventilation and, therefore, by exercise (Hawkins 1976), with a half-life of 2 hours during exercise and as long as 8–10 hours during sleep (Castleden and Cole 1974). Thus, carbon monoxide may reach a "nonsmoking" cut point in 6–24 hours in a person who smokes regularly depending on their activity, and people who smoke less often per day or smoke only intermittently will often have an eCO level below 6 ppm.

Because portable carbon monoxide monitors are widely available and can be used to assess recent smoke exposure or to biochemically confirm smoking cessation (e.g., eCO <6 ppm) and provide direct feedback to patients in minutes, they are an essential tool for any clinical practice that is serious about helping its patients quit smoking, in much the same way a blood pressure measurement via a sphygmomanometer is a standard part of any medical assessment (Benowitz et al. 2020). With the advent of new technology and the acceptance of "remote" clinical practice (particularly during the worldwide coronavirus disease 2019 [COVID-19] pandemic), personal eCO monitors are now available for single-person use that may boost individuals' motivation to quit (Marler et al. 2020) and enable biochemical assessment during remote smoking cessation treatment (Tuck et al. 2021)

Assessment Summary

Although the variety of assessment tools and potential nicotine products may appear somewhat bewildering, in clinical practice each of the following questions, either on their own or when added together, will provide a fairly clear indication of how addicted a nicotine user is:

1. How many days out of the past 30 did you use your tobacco product? _____ (>19)
2. How many times per day do you usually use your tobacco product? _____ (>4)
3. On days that you can use your tobacco product freely, how soon after you wake up do you first use your tobacco product (in minutes)? _____ (<30)
4. How addicted would you say you are to your tobacco product? (a) Not at all addicted (b) somewhat addicted (c) very addicted _____ (> not at all)

Any nicotine product user who uses their product on 20 or more days out of 30, uses at least four times per day, uses within the first 30 minutes of waking in the morning, or believes that they are somewhat or very addicted to their product should be regarded as likely meeting criteria for addiction, dependence, or TUD and likely requiring treatment to increase their chances of successfully quitting in the long term.

Assessing Nicotine Withdrawal

As described in Chapter 3, when a regular nicotine user abruptly abstains or markedly reduces consumption, they are likely to experience an increase in a group of symptoms that have consistently been demonstrated to be caused specifically by nicotine withdrawal (i.e., in the sense that they are relieved by nicotine replacement therapy in double-blind trials). It is good practice when assessing a tobacco user prior to treatment to assess these symptoms at baseline while the person is still using and then to assess again at later time points during treatment to help decide which symptoms are abstinence-related and to guide the dosage of medications that can be used to reduce withdrawal symptom severity.

By far the most widely used and fully validated assessment tool for assessing nicotine withdrawal is the Minnesota Tobacco Withdrawal

Scale (MTWS; Table 4–5) (Hughes and Hatsukami 1986). Although the wording may be changed slightly (e.g., with regard to the time frame of the questions), the most widely used wording is shown in the table. Note that if a heading is used for this assessment, the recommendation is to simply call it a "behavior rating scale" to encourage participants to simply rate how they are feeling, rather than to make judgments as to the cause.

The score from the first eight items can be summed to create a total score. Specific items that were low at baseline and "severe" after quitting tobacco may require attention, particularly for individuals with a history of having difficulties managing those types of emotions (e.g., anger, depression, eating disorders) or for whom a marked worsening could have serious implications in their life circumstances (e.g., an air traffic controller who is having difficulty concentrating). Regular assessment of these symptoms also may be used to guide the need for nicotine replacement therapy for individuals who are required to comply with nicotine abstinence because of their residential circumstances (e.g., patients admitted to a hospital, inmates admitted to prison or jail, hospital staff on a long shift).

Table 4–5. Minnesota Tobacco Withdrawal Scale

Please rate yourself for the last 24 hours. 0 = none, 1 = slight, 2 = mild, 3 = moderate, 4 = severe.

Angry, irritable, frustrated	0	1	2	3	4
Anxious, nervous	0	1	2	3	4
Depressed mood, sad	0	1	2	3	4
Difficulty concentrating	0	1	2	3	4
Increased appetite, hungry, weight gain	0	1	2	3	4
Insomnia, sleep problems, awakening at night	0	1	2	3	4
Restless	0	1	2	3	4
Impatient	0	1	2	3	4
Craving to smoke	0	1	2	3	4

Source. Hughes and Hatsukami 1986.

Assessing Motivation to Quit or Reduce Tobacco/Nicotine Use

In addition to assessing tobacco use and the severity of the patient's addiction to nicotine/tobacco products, the other key component of the evaluation is assessing their level of interest in changing their tobacco use behavior. One of the most widely used models of behavior change is typically described as the "Stages of Change" model, which asks participants to select which statement best describes their recent or current interest in quitting smoking (DiClemente et al. 1991):

- Are you seriously thinking about quitting smoking in the next 6 months?
- Do you have a specific plan to quit smoking in the next 30 days?
- Have you made a serious attempt to stop smoking in the past 12 months that lasted for at least 1 week and was not because you were in the hospital?
- Have you made an attempt to quit smoking in the past 6 months and are still trying to stay quit?

People in the *precontemplation* stage are not thinking of quitting smoking in the next 6 months. Those in the *contemplation* stage are "seriously thinking about quitting smoking in the next 2–6 months" but either are not planning to do so in the next month or have not made a serious attempt to quit in the past year that lasted at least 1 week. The *preparation* stage refers to people who have a specific plan to quit smoking in the next month and have made at least one serious attempt to quit in the past year that lasted at least 1 week. People in the *action* stage have been trying to quit or maintain abstinence during the past 6 months and are still trying (with some relapses). When a person reaches the *maintenance* stage, they have successfully quit smoking for longer than 6 months. The Transtheoretical Model of Behavior Change (Prochaska et al. 1994) proposed that it is helpful to assess each person's stage of change and to deliver a stage-specific intervention to help them move in a positive direction toward long-term tobacco abstinence (maintenance). The Stages of Change model has intuitive appeal to practitioners, but strict interpretation of it has been criticized on various grounds, including that it does not reflect the observation that people sometimes change their behavior and plans quite suddenly and sometimes in response to seemingly small triggers (West 2005). For example, studies have found that surprisingly large proportions of quit attempts involve little to no planning at all (Larabie 2005), and other studies have found considerable instability in intentions to quit smoking over short periods. The main concerns with the Stages of Change assessment are that it may prevent potentially important interventions from being offered to people who are in precontemplation (e.g., because they feel they are too addicted to quit) and that it may give practitioners a false sense that progress is being made when patients are encouraged to begin thinking about quitting, when in reality very little has meaningfully changed.

There are numerous other methods of assessing motivation to quit tobacco use, with the simplest ones being to ask about desire, likelihood, and confidence (also called "self-efficacy"):

1. How much do you want to stop smoking? (a) Not at all (b) Somewhat (c) Very much
2. How likely is it that you will stop smoking in the next month? (a) Not likely (b) Somewhat likely (c) Very likely
3. How confident are you that you will succeed in stopping smoking in the next month? (a) Not at all confident (b) Somewhat confident (c) Very confident

Each of these types of assessment has their uses, with the most basic being that they identify which tobacco users are already highly motivated to move directly into a quit attempt and which may benefit from additional encouragement, support, and motivation to make changes. Simply from a perspective of respecting the personal autonomy of others, it is clear that a person who smokes and is in the precontemplation stage is unlikely to respond well if they are simply told that they must quit smoking and handed a prescription for a smoking cessation medicine. Methods that can be successful in stimulating quit attempts and increasing the chances of successfully quitting are discussed in subsequent chapters.

Case Example

Roberto (age 43) is a computer programmer who smokes 10 CPD, with the first of the day being 60 minutes after waking in the morning, when he gets in his car to drive to work. His wife has never allowed smoking in the home because one of their children has asthma. His workplace does not allow smoking in the office, and he has little opportunity to leave for more than three short breaks. He has never tried to quit smoking, and over the past 2 years he has started to supplement his smoking by using oral nicotine pouches at times when he cannot leave the office for a smoke break (three to five times per day). However, an older colleague who smokes recently had a heart attack, so Roberto has become more interested in quitting. His FTCD score is low because of his fairly low cigarette consumption and long time to first cigarette.

What Are the Concerns in This Case?

Roberto is an example of someone for whom it is not simple to verify their difficulty quitting or strong withdrawal symptoms when quitting because he has never seriously tried to quit. However, around 80% of people who smoke 10 CPD meet DSM-5 criteria for TUD and, on average, meet 4 of the 11 criteria, which indicates "moderate" dependence. The fact that Roberto is supplementing with oral nicotine pouches also strongly indicates that he is likely to be at least moderately dependent. When considering pharmacotherapy, there are no apparent reasons to consider starting him on anything other than a full dose.

Key Points

- When assessing nicotine dependence, it is important to ask patients about use of any nicotine products, not just cigarettes or the product they use most frequently.
- Most people who have smoked on 20 or more days out of the past 30 days are at least mildly dependent, and although other nicotine products may not be equally as addictive as cigarettes, daily use is a strong indicator of dependence.
- The other key signs of stronger dependence are 1) frequent product use and 2) experiences of craving and withdrawal during abstinence.
- People with higher dependence are less likely to quit and are more likely to benefit from pharmacotherapy and behavioral support.

References

American Psychiatric Association: Diagnostic and Statistical Manual of Mental Disorders, 4th Edition. Washington, DC, American Psychiatric Association, 1994

American Psychiatric Association: Diagnostic and Statistical Manual of Mental Disorders, 5th Edition, Text Revision. Washington, DC, American Psychiatric Association, 2022

Baker TB, Breslau N, Covey L, et al: DSM criteria for tobacco use disorder and tobacco withdrawal: a critique and proposed revisions for DSM-5. Addiction 107(2):263–275, 2012 21919989

Benowitz NL, Bernert JT, Foulds J, et al: Biochemical verification of tobacco use and abstinence: 2019 update. Nicotine Tob Res 22(7):1086–1097, 2020 31570931

Bover MT, Foulds J, Steinberg MB, et al: Waking at night to smoke as a marker for tobacco dependence: patient characteristics and relationship to treatment outcome. Int J Clin Pract 62(2):182–190, 2008 18199277

Brook JS, Koppel J, Pahl K: Predictors of DSM and Fagerström-defined nicotine dependence in African American and Puerto Rican young adults. Subst Use Misuse 44(6):809–822, 2009 19444723

Caraballo RS, Holiday DB, Stellman SD, et al: Comparison of serum cotinine concentration within and across smokers of menthol and nonmenthol cigarette brands among non-Hispanic black and non-Hispanic white U.S. adult smokers, 2001–2006. Cancer Epidemiol Biomarkers Prev 20(7):1329–1340, 2011 21430301

Castleden CM, Cole PV: Variations in carboxyhaemoglobin levels in smokers. BMJ 4(5947):736–738, 1974 4441877

DiClemente CC, Prochaska JO, Fairhurst SK, et al: The process of smoking cessation: an analysis of precontemplation, contemplation, and preparation stages of change. J Consult Clin Psychol 59(2):295–304, 1991 2030191

DiFranza JR, Savageau JA, Fletcher K, et al: Measuring the loss of autonomy over nicotine use in adolescents: the DANDY (Development and Assessment of Nicotine Dependence in Youths) study. Arch Pediatr Adolesc Med 156(4):397–403, 2002 11929376

DiFranza JR, Wellman RJ, Savageau JA, et al: What aspect of dependence does the Fagerström Test for Nicotine Dependence measure? ISRN Addict 2013:906276, 2012 25969829

Fagerström K, Russ C, Yu C-R, et al: The Fagerström Test for Nicotine Dependence as a predictor of smoking abstinence: a pooled analysis of varenicline clinical trial data. Nicotine Tob Res 14(12):1467–1473, 2012 22467778

Fidler JA, West R: Enjoyment of smoking and urges to smoke as predictors of attempts and success of attempts to stop smoking: a longitudinal study. Drug Alcohol Depend 115(1–2):30–34, 2011 21111539

Fiore MC, Adsit R: Will hospitals finally "do the right thing"? Providing evidence-based tobacco dependence treatments to hospitalized patients who smoke. Jt Comm J Qual Patient Saf 42(5):207–208, 2016 27066923

Foulds J, Veldheer S, Hrabovsky S, et al: The effect of motivational lung age feedback on short-term quit rates in smokers seeking intensive group treatment: a randomized controlled pilot study. Drug Alcohol Depend 153:271–277, 2015a 26051163

Foulds J, Veldheer S, Yingst J, et al: Development of a questionnaire for assessing dependence on electronic cigarettes among a large sample of ex-smoking e-cigarette users. Nicotine Tob Res 17(2):186–192, 2015b 25332459

Hawkins LH: Blood carbon monoxide levels as a function of daily cigarette consumption and physical activity. Br J Ind Med 33(2):123–125, 1976 1276092

Heatherton TF, Kozlowski LT, Frecker RC, et al: Measuring the heaviness of smoking: using self-reported time to the first cigarette of the day and number of cigarettes smoked per day. Br J Addict 84(7):791–799, 1989 2758152

Heatherton TF, Kozlowski LT, Frecker RC, et al: The Fagerström Test for Nicotine Dependence: a revision of the Fagerström Tolerance Questionnaire. Br J Addict 86(9):1119–1127, 1991 1932883

Holford TR, McKay L, Jeon J, et al: Smoking histories by state in the U.S. Am J Prev Med 64(4 Suppl 1):S42–S52, 2023 36653233

Hughes JR, Hatsukami D: Signs and symptoms of tobacco withdrawal. Arch Gen Psychiatry 43(3):289–294, 1986 3954551

Jarvis MJ, Belcher M, Vesey C, et al: Low cost carbon monoxide monitors in smoking assessment. Thorax 41(11):886–887, 1986 3824275

Larabie LC: To what extent do smokers plan quit attempts? Tob Control 14(6):425–428, 2005 16319368

Liu Y, Pan IE, Tak HJ, et al: Assessment of uptake appropriateness of computed tomography for lung cancer screening according to patients meeting eligibility criteria of the US Preventive Services Task Force. JAMA Netw Open 5(11):e2243163, 2022 36409492

Marler JD, Fujii CA, Wong KS, et al: Assessment of a personal interactive carbon monoxide breath sensor in people who smoke cigarettes: single-arm cohort study. J Med Internet Res 22(10):e22811, 2020 32894829

Moolchan ET, Zimmerman D, Sehnert SS, et al: Recent marijuana blunt smoking impacts carbon monoxide as a measure of adolescent tobacco abstinence. Subst Use Misuse 40(2):231–240, 2005 15770886

Morean ME, Krishnan-Sarin S, Sussman S, et al: Psychometric evaluation of the e-cigarette dependence scale. Nicotine Tob Res 21(11):1556–1564, 2019 29301008

Mushtaq N, Beebe LA: Psychometric properties of Fagerström Test for Nicotine Dependence for Smokeless Tobacco Users (FTND-ST). Nicotine Tob Res 19(9):1095–1101, 2017 28387864

Oliver JA, Foulds J: Association between cigarette smoking frequency and tobacco use disorder in U.S. adults. Am J Prev Med 60(5):726–728, 2021 33358276

Pienkowski M, Chaiton M, Dubray J, et al: E-cigarette dependence in youth. Nicotine Tob Res 24(7):1089–1094, 2022 34936704

Piper ME, Baker TB, Benowitz NL, et al: E-cigarette dependence measures in dual users: reliability and relations with dependence criteria and e-cigarette cessation. Nicotine Tob Res 22(5):756–763, 2020 30874804

Pokhrel P, Kawamoto CT, Mettias H, et al: Predictors of discontinued e-cigarette use at one-year follow-up in a sample of young adults. Int J Environ Res Public Health 20(6):4770, 2023 36981678

Prochaska JO, Velicer WF, Rossi JS, et al: Stages of change and decisional balance for 12 problem behaviors. Health Psychol 13(1):39–46, 1994 8168470

Shiffman S: How many cigarettes did you smoke? Assessing cigarette consumption by global report, time-line follow-back, and ecological momentary assessment. Health Psychol 28(5):519–526, 2009 19751076

Shiffman S, Scholl SM, Mao J, et al: Using nicotine gum to assist nondaily smokers in quitting: a randomized clinical trial. Nicotine Tob Res 22(3):390–397, 2020 31125988

Sobieski E, Yingst J, Foulds J: Quitting electronic cigarettes: factors associated with quitting and quit attempts in long-term users. Addict Behav 127:107220, 2022 34979427

Tindle HA, Shiffman S: Smoking cessation behavior among intermittent smokers versus daily smokers. Am J Public Health 101(7):e1–e3, 2011 21566030

Tual S, Piau J-P, Jarvis MJ, et al: Impact of tobacco control policies on exhaled carbon monoxide in non-smokers. J Epidemiol Community Health 64(6):554–556, 2010 20466721

Tuck BM, Karelitz JL, Tomko RL, et al: Mobile, remote, and individual focused: comparing breath carbon monoxide readings and abstinence between smartphone-enabled and stand-alone monitors. Nicotine Tob Res 23(4):741–747, 2021 33022057

Van Overmeire IPI, De Smedt T, Dendale P, et al: Nicotine dependence and urinary nicotine, cotinine and hydroxycotinine levels in daily smokers. Nicotine Tob Res 18(9):1813–1819, 2016 27083213

Wellman RJ, Savageau JA, Godiwala S, et al: A comparison of the Hooked on Nicotine Checklist and the Fagerström Test for Nicotine Dependence in adult smokers. Nicotine Tob Res 8(4):575–580, 2006 16920655

West R: Time for a change: putting the transtheoretical (stages of change) model to rest. Addiction 100(8):1036–1039, 2005 16042624

Yingst J, Wang X, Lopez AA, et al: Changes in nicotine dependence among smokers using electronic cigarettes to reduce cigarette smoking in a randomized controlled trial. Nicotine Tob Res 25(3):372–378, 2023 35752091

5

Tobacco Comorbidity With Other Behavioral Health Conditions

Smoking rates are at an all-time low in the United States, largely due to decades of successful tobacco control efforts. These public health initiatives have dramatically changed the public view of tobacco, leading to fewer people starting to use tobacco products and more people successfully quitting. Components of this approach include increased tobacco taxes, antismoking advertisements, age restrictions on tobacco purchases, tobacco-free air laws, and policies that restrict use in public places and workplaces, as well as support for tobacco cessation treatments. Even in recent decades, the proportion of U.S. adults who smoke cigarettes continues to decline (from 20.9% in 2005 to 13.7% in 2018) (Jamal et al. 2018); however, important disparities in cigarette smoking persist. Tobacco use rates remain high among several disadvantaged and marginalized populations, notably those with lower socioeconomic status as measured by income, education, or access to health insurance. Cigarette smoking rates are higher among males, Native Americans, and people who have lower education, have low income, or were uninsured or insured through Medicaid (Jamal et al. 2018). M0uch higher tobacco use rates also are seen among military veterans, individuals with a disability, or those who identify as lesbian, gay, or bisexual (Odani et al. 2018). Some of the highest rates of smoking are found among individuals who report having a mental illness or another substance use disorder (SUD); these rates are at least double those seen in people without these disorders. This pattern has persisted since the early 2000s and is worsened by factors such as poverty (Centers for Disease Control and Prevention 2023; Lawrence et al. 2009; National Center for Health Statistics 2017; Office of the Surgeon General 2020). This disparity was highlighted in the 2020 Surgeon General's Report (Figure 5–1).

Although there is encouraging evidence that tobacco use rates have declined somewhat in this group in recent decades, they are declining at a slower rate than in other populations (Han et al. 2022; Weinberger et al. 2020). In the United States, quit rates among individuals with past-month serious psychological distress (SPD), a proxy measurement for serious mental illness, are approximately half the quit rates of those without SPD, and they have not increased in recent decades (Streck et al. 2020). Some studies have estimated that individuals with current mental illness or SUD make up at least one-third of people in the

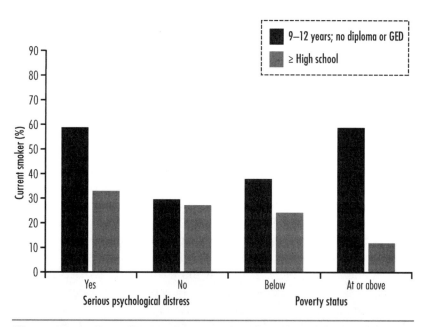

Figure 5–1. Prevalence of current cigarette smoking by level of education and presence or absence of serious psychological distress and poverty status among adults 25 years of age and older.
GED = general educational development.

Source. National Center for Health Statistics 2017; Office of the Surgeon General 2020.

United States who currently smoke and purchase at least one-third of all tobacco products (Grant et al. 2004; Office of the Surgeon General 2020; Streck et al. 2020).

Although high tobacco use rates were originally reported only in clinical samples of individuals receiving some type of behavioral health services, these findings have been validated across many nationally representative and broader population studies. This includes state, national, and even international data, suggesting these high rates are a worldwide phenomenon, at least for developed nations (de Leon and Diaz 2005; Guydish et al. 2016; Lawrence et al. 2009). Higher tobacco use rates are associated with nearly every specific mental illness diagnostic group, including anxiety disorders, mood disorders, psychotic disorders, ADHD, and SUDs (Smith et al. 2014b). Among people with a behavioral health condition, smoking rates are higher in those receiving mental health treatment, with a lifetime smoking prevalence of 60% (Smith et al. 2014b). Because many of these mental health conditions are common, with lifetime prevalence rates of 20%–40%, and individuals can meet criteria for multiple disorders, this finding underscores the large numbers involved and the tremendous overlap of these comorbid groups.

Data from the National Epidemiologic Survey on Alcohol and Related Conditions (NESARC) that include DSM diagnoses indicate that individuals with any current psychiatric diagnosis had 3.2 times greater odds of currently smoking than those with no diagnosis and were 25% less likely to have quit by follow-up (Smith et al. 2014b). Having multiple diagnoses was also associated with a greater likelihood of smoking heavily (Smith et al. 2014b). Prevalence varied by specific diagnoses, as did cessation rates. Because some disorders are more challenging to measure in household surveys, with many false-positives (e.g., psychotic disorders), estimates of serious mental illness are conducted in many epidemiological studies. The best-known is the K6, a six-item scale that measures SPD (Kessler et al. 2002). Although the K6 is nonspecific, it has been clinically validated, has been consistently shown to be associated with higher tobacco use rates, and can be used to track trends over time.

Tobacco use rates are similarly higher in populations with alcohol use disorder or other SUDs. Clinical and epidemiological studies reveal that smoking use in these populations occurs at rates two to four times higher than in other groups (Guydish et al. 2016). Again, clinical overlap and comorbidity are the rule. SPD is more than twice as common among adults with SUD who smoke cigarettes compared with those without SUD who do not smoke cigarettes (Parker et al. 2021).

Why Higher Rates?

Reasons for the strong co-occurrence are not known. Multiple vulnerabilities may lead to this disparity and include a range of biopsychosocial factors. Evidence suggests that having a mental illness is associated with an increased vulnerability to develop daily smoking and tobacco use disorder (TUD). The opposite is also true. Tobacco use as a young person seems to be a biological marker that predicts not only the presence but also the severity of subsequent mental illness. These factors can lead to higher rates of smoking initiation and progression to daily smoking and can also be important barriers to cessation. A shared biological or genetic predisposition is certainly possible. All mental illnesses share an increased risk for developing an SUD, among which TUD is included. Psychological factors can include impaired coping strategies and a sense of hopelessness, as well as low confidence in being able to quit. Using tobacco (or other substances) to cope with the profound effects of mental illness, or the boredom and isolation that may result, is commonly reported. Although specific examples are included in each subsection that follows, many of these concepts cross domains and do not fit into discrete biological, psychological, or social categories. The experience of craving or urges to use tobacco, for example, can be conceptualized as a phenomenon that is at the same time biological, psychological, and mediated by social factors. For our purposes here, it is included in the psychological domain.

Biological Vulnerability

Having a mental health problem at a young age is associated with a higher risk of being a tobacco user. Many diagnoses are linked to smoking in youth, including mood and anxiety disorders, ADHD, and other SUDs. Nicotine is known to modulate the brain circuits that are disturbed in these disorders, and the same risks are presumed with electronic (e-)cigarettes or vaping nicotine (Becker et al. 2021). There is concern that e-cigarette use in youth will increase the subsequent risk for smoking traditional cigarettes. Brain development and myelination are not completed until about the age of 25; therefore, youth have an increased vulnerability to the effects of substances, particularly in the frontal lobe, which is essential for judgment, reasoning, and problem-solving. Nicotine's effects on these processes are not well understood. Individuals with mental illness have an increased vulnerability to TUD in terms of the progression of smoking. Youth with behavioral health problems are more likely to progress to daily use and addiction to nicotine (Breslau et al. 2004; U.S. Department of Health and Human Services 2012). Attention and hyperactivity symptoms are linked to an increased odds of ever smoking, early initiation of smoking in children and adolescents, and a greater progression to regular smoking (Charach et al. 2011; Gray and Upadhyaya 2009; Mitchell et al. 2019).

For years, it was believed that smoking lessened the symptoms of mental illness, the so-called self-medication hypothesis. In many cases, this was overstated and may have even been propagated by the tobacco industry as a way to legitimize smoking in vulnerable populations (Prochaska et al. 2008). Nicotine clearly has an impact on attention and concentration, and studies link a possible benefit in ADHD. For other conditions, the data are less clear. In schizophrenia, heavy nicotine use has been linked with a possible benefit in impaired working memory systems when measured in a laboratory setting, although the clinical benefit of this is less clear. Any possible benefits from nicotine do not outweigh the considerable harms associated with tobacco and smoke exposure and are never a rationale for smoking, although they could support the continued use of nicotine medication. An alternative to the self-medication hypothesis is that developmental changes that lead to mental illness are linked to strong biological vulnerabilities for SUDs (Berg et al. 2014) and that this shared biology is the real reason for high comorbidities with tobacco. For example, evidence from animal and human studies implicates adult hippocampal neurogenesis in the pathophysiology of substance addiction and mental illness. Animal studies show that addictive substances, including nicotine, reduce hippocampal neurogenic activity, which may help explain how addictive substance use typically worsens rather than improves psychiatric syndromes and lends support to arguments that dual-diagnosis disorders represent disease synergies rather than merely "self-medication" (Chambers 2013).

Populations with other SUDs have among the highest rates of tobacco use, and comorbidity is the rule because people do not generally restrict their use of substances to only one. Relationships of tobacco use to nearly every form of other substance use, including alcohol, cannabis, and opioids, are well documented. In youth, tobacco is often the first substance used, although it is closely timed around the first use of alcohol and cannabis. Vulnerability factors are also linked and over-lapping. In college populations, use of alcohol and tobacco is highly correlated and often shows patterns of weekly use centered around the weekend.

There is now considerable evidence that those with a behavioral health condition (mental illness or SUD) have higher levels of addiction to tobacco (also called TUD severity in DSM-5 nomenclature [American Psychiatric Association 2022]) than those without. This can be quantified as using more tobacco per day (typically measured as cigarettes per day). Heavy smoking is also more common. The faster time to first cigarette smoked in the morning, a well-validated measure of TUD severity, is also seen in populations with mental illness (Hagman et al. 2008; Pratt and Brody 2010).

Populations with behavioral health comorbidity also experience more difficulty quitting tobacco, both in a given attempt and over their lifetime. This has been shown in large clinical trials and population studies (Glasheen et al. 2014; Hagman et al. 2008; Smith et al. 2014b). National declines in smoking are not being realized to the same extent among people with mental illness (Cook et al. 2014). This can be linked not only to higher levels of dependence but also to other biopsychosocial factors, such as poor coping and low self-efficacy. It also suggests that tobacco control policies and environmental strategies have not worked as effectively for this population because many facilities continue to allow smoking on the behavioral health treatment grounds and have been slow to adopt on-site treatment. There is also some evidence of reduced success with attempts to quit among this population when compared with people who smoke but do not have a mental illness in similar conditions (Anthenelli et al. 2016).

There is also evidence of higher levels of tobacco withdrawal and craving in people with mental illness who smoke, making it more challenging to quit and supporting the need for intensive treatments and more pharmacotherapies (Piper et al. 2011; Weinberger et al. 2010). Population data have also shown a substantially greater likelihood of nicotine withdrawal in people with mental illness, which contributes to considerable distress and undermines quit attempts, despite motivation (Smith et al. 2014a). Advances in understanding the biology of addiction reveal the importance not only of dopaminergic reward pathways but also of the extended amygdala and its role in processes of withdrawal and distress coping. Relief of negative affect, whether it is caused by substance withdrawal, negative mood states, or other factors that manifest as distress, is a driving force in seeking and using substances, including nicotine. This is discussed in more detail in the "Psychological Factors" section that follows. Stress, trauma, and substance use are strongly linked, and the stress response is linked to substance initiation, maintenance, and relapse. Although stress may influence the use of substances as a way to cope or relieve distress, substance use also seems to activate hypothalamic-pituitary and sympathetic nervous systems pathways that induce stress (Lemieux and al'Absi 2016).

Shared biological mechanisms among individuals with SUD could impact craving and relapse. Nicotine can enhance the rewarding effects of other substances. Withdrawal symptoms are often nonspecific and can be overlapping. Some tobacco use may be intended to lessen symptoms of withdrawal from other substances.

Psychological Factors

Psychological factors related to tobacco use are numerous and can include attitudes about quitting, smoking in order to cope, or managing negative moods or subjective distress. Although these are discussed as discrete categories, blurring occurs between biological and psychological factors in many areas. Beliefs about smoking as well as about quitting are important to determine because they predict whether the person will decide to continue smoking on the basis of their risk versus benefit assessment. Across qualitative studies, relief of distress, social inclusion, and mental health symptom management appear to be highly important beliefs for smoking among people with serious mental illness (Trainor and Leavey 2017). Quitting for health benefits and financial savings, although important, is rated as less important by this group than the perceived benefits of smoking. Despite barriers, many studies have shown that people with mental illness—even serious mental illness—who smoke are as or perhaps even more motivated to try to quit as others who smoke (Siru et al. 2009). Beliefs that quitting will worsen their mental health symptoms or cause recurrence or relapse are common barriers in those with mental illness or SUD. These are discussed in more detail in Chapter 11.

Great advances have also been made in understanding addiction and substance-seeking behaviors, even in the context of continued use despite consequences. Behaviors are thought to shift from the impulsive to the compulsive as substance use progresses and becomes more problematic. Rather than use substances for pleasure (termed *positive reinforcement* or *reward*), they develop alternative drives. These are tied to learning behaviors and are termed *negative reinforcement* (Kassel et al. 2003). Negative reinforcement contributes to much drug-seeking behavior and substance use because it implies that using substances will reduce or eliminate bad feelings or distress. One example of negative reinforcement is using substances to take away the uncomfortable symptoms of withdrawal. Tobacco users often experience withdrawal every morning because nicotine has a short half-life and disappears from the body during sleep. This contributes to morning smoking to alleviate withdrawal symptoms, which can interfere with successfully quitting. Negative reinforcement can be generalized to any feelings of sadness or distress, including depression, anxiety, and other mental health symptoms, that are relieved by substance use. A history of trauma or the presence of social factors such as poverty or social deprivation might be factors that drive continued substance use to cope with uncomfortable or overwhelming feelings.

Among substance users, many behaviors may be shared that also impact the craving or use of tobacco. This may be especially true if the person also smokes other substances. Recent studies show that the rise in daily cannabis users in recent decades is almost entirely in individuals who also smoke tobacco (Goodwin et al. 2018). Being a cannabis user is associated with less success in quitting smoking, and quit ratios are lower among this population. Tobacco users may be trying to cope with various negative mood states as well as with boredom or cravings for other substances.

Rather than focus on clinical diagnoses, which have considerable variability, it may be more useful to look at processes that underlie and contribute to many mental illnesses. This transdiagnostic approach proposes that certain dimensions, traits, neural circuits, and biological pathways that are shared across mental disorder diagnoses can have more predictive value than diagnostic categories (Cuthbert and Insel 2013). Leventhal and Zvolensky (2015) proposed a novel framework for understanding the complex interactions of mental health symptoms, including depression and anxiety, on smoking. They described three vulnerabilities—anhedonia, anxiety sensitivity, and distress tolerance—that underpin many diagnoses, promote smoking behaviors, and interfere with cessation. This model suggests that individuals with mental health conditions have an increased vulnerability to the effects of smoking (or other substance use), at least in part because they have a maladaptive response to emotional states and stronger-than-usual beliefs (expectancies) that smoking will help. Although discussed as discrete domains, these likely overlap, with interacting relationships that can be more severe and challenging to overcome.

Anhedonia

Anhedonia describes a state of deficient enjoyment or pleasure in things that are commonly rewarding or enjoyable. It can be a characteristic of depression as well as of other disorders, such as schizophrenia, and can be somewhat stable over time, leading to behavioral withdrawal or decreased motivation. With anhedonia, only high-potency rewards, such as smoking (or other substance use), may elicit a positive hedonic response and enhance the reinforcing properties of the substance. Chronically, reliance on the substance may increase in order to maintain this hedonic tone. These individuals could be more sensitive to the negative mood effects of tobacco withdrawal, leading to more relapses (Leventhal and Zvolensky 2015).

Anxiety Sensitivity

Anxiety sensitivity refers to fears and negative beliefs that anxiety symptoms or feelings will be intolerable and are a sign of imminent danger. This can lead to maladaptive coping, avoidance behaviors, and negative emotional states. Although smoking and nicotine use over time generally increase anxiety, someone with anxiety sensitivity may rely on smoking to manage anxiety states and body sensations, creating a vicious circle that is hard to disrupt. These individuals may be fearful about attempting to quit smoking and often experience worse tobacco withdrawal symptoms (which includes feeling anxious) and more relapses during stressful situations (Audrain-McGovern et al. 2015; Leventhal and Zvolensky 2015).

Distress Tolerance

Distress tolerance describes the ability to withstand and tolerate negative (emotional or other) states, including frustration, pain, or stress. Personality disorders, as well as anxiety, eating disorders, and SUDs, are all associated with worse distress tolerance. Individuals with low tolerance often use low-effort coping skills (e.g., eating or using substances) to manage and reduce distress. These behaviors can undermine a long-term goal, such as quitting smoking, in lieu of immediate relief. A related idea of *task persistence*, or being able to endure uncomfortable feelings to complete a task, is associated with more success when attempting to quit.

Social and Environmental Factors

Many social factors are linked with a higher risk for smoking and greater challenges to quitting. Lower socioeconomic status, as measured by lower levels of education, lower income, and reduced or lack of access to health insurance, is consistently associated with higher tobacco use. As smoking rates have decreased in the U.S. general population, smoking has become more concentrated in these disadvantaged groups. This multitude of factors also includes social identities of race and ethnicity, sex, and gender identity, which interact with each other and have multilevel effects. How these interact with other societal factors, including discrimination, societal trauma, and stigma, becomes quite complex. The combined effects or intersectionality can be greater than the effects of a single factor and can have numerous negative psychological effects on individuals, which can, in turn, influence smoking and substance use behaviors (Sheffer et al. 2022). We must understand these complexities to avoid reducing people to single categories and to better tailor our approaches and work with individuals with complex disparities. This understanding may be essential for overcoming health disparities because people are members of different groups simultaneously, and these factors can cluster together to worsen outcomes.

These social factors are important and contribute to smoking initiation, progression, and likelihood of successfully quitting. The influence of peers is seen not only among youth, and this modeling behavior can influence others through active or passive processes. Even among people with mental illness, having family or peers who express negative views about tobacco and having nonsmoking family and friends are associated with more intent to quit and greater use of tobacco treatment medications (Nagawa et al. 2022).

Tobacco-free policies that restrict smoking in the workplace or residential environment have been highly effective in reducing tobacco use in the United States, both by encouraging cessation and by contributing to reduced use among youth. Populations with behavioral health comorbidity, like other low-income populations, may be less affected by environmental tobacco restrictions if they are not in the workforce or if their worksite is less likely to have such restrictions (Delnevo et al. 2004).

Targeted marketing by the tobacco industry has been very effective in shaping norms around tobacco use. It targets marketing to populations that include young adults, socially disadvantaged groups, and various racial and ethnic groups. Industry strategies include brand creation; advertising imagery and placement, including the presence of more tobacco advertisements and billboards in neighborhoods with diverse populations and lower socioeconomic status; event sponsorships; and promotional items. The tobacco industry segments consumer markets into groups such as those who smoke to fill a psychological need (e.g., stress relief, behavioral arousal, performance enhancement, obesity reduction) and—as more recent evidence has revealed—those who are psychologically vulnerable, including the mentally ill (Apollonio and Malone 2005). Until recently, most psychiatric hospitals sold cigarettes in the hospital store, which meant that they received frequent sales promotions and giveaways from major cigarette companies promoting value brands. The industry also supported efforts to block smoking bans in these settings.

Among people who receive services within the behavioral health system, there is a culture that, in the past, endorsed the use of tobacco. Although the system has moved away from using tobacco as an explicit reward, an attitude of ambivalence about addressing its use as an addiction has too often persisted. Thus, systems have been slow to change and to keep up with innovations in evidence-based treatments and tobacco-free policies. Rates of assessment and treatment for tobacco use remain low in these settings. Psychiatrists are less likely to be aware of and to implement cessation resources and practice guidelines (Young et al. 2023). Mental health and substance abuse clinicians continue to endorse negative beliefs about addressing tobacco that delay progress, including that tobacco is less harmful than other substances; they believe it is not their job to treat tobacco use and that such treatment will only harm patients (Hunt et al. 2014). Tobacco treatment practices actually appeared to decline among psychiatrists over a 15-year period (Rogers and Sherman 2014), which may be a result of staffing issues and competing priorities as psychiatric provider shortages continue to worsen. Despite these challenges, patients are interested in treatment, and staff should be supported to deliver integrated treatment for tobacco use in behavioral health treatment settings. Strategies for addressing systems change in behavioral health treatment settings are discussed in Chapter 10.

Consequences of Tobacco Use

As reviewed in Chapter 1, smoke from burning cigarettes is estimated to contain thousands of different chemical components, more than 65 of which are known to be carcinogenic. The negative effects of products of combustion, including carbon monoxide, on cardiovascular health are well documented. Although nicotine is responsible for the addiction to tobacco, it does not cause the numerous cancers and other chronic diseases attributed to the other chemicals found in tobacco and smoke. Not surprisingly, tobacco use is the number one cause of death among mental health (Callaghan et al. 2014) and substance-using populations, surpassing even deaths due to the use of alcohol or other substances (Hurt et al. 1996; Veldhuizen and Callaghan 2014). Helping patients stop smoking is the most important approach to preventing cardiovascular disease and metabolic syndrome (Correll 2007; Rogers and Sherman 2014). Among people with SPD, smoking doubles the risk of death (Tam et al. 2016). Individuals with mental illness or SUD have worse health outcomes on nearly every measure, and tobacco use is a main risk factor for many comorbid medical conditions. Many studies have shown reduced life expectancy in these groups, with 50% of deaths attributable to diseases caused by tobacco (Bandiera et al. 2015; Callaghan et al. 2014). In people with schizophrenia, cigarette smoking increases the cardiovascular mortality rate significantly over the life span (by 86% over 20 years) (Stolz et al. 2019).

Smoking or having smoked cigarettes in the past increases the risk of severe illness due to coronavirus disease 2019 (COVID-19) for numerous potential reasons, including that smoking compromises immune function and is associated with more comorbidities that increase COVID-19 risk, such as cardiovascular diseases and chronic obstructive pulmonary disease (Centers for Disease Control and Prevention 2023). In addition to the health consequences, tobacco use also threatens recovery for these individuals by impacting them negatively in finances, employability, and housing (Houle and Siegel 2009; Steinberg et al. 2004). Low-income populations spend at least 25% of their monthly income on cigarettes (Farrelly et al. 2012; Steinberg et al. 2004). People with a mental disorder or SUD are estimated to purchase and consume 30%–44% of all cigarettes sold, making them a sizable percentage of the U.S. tobacco market (Grant et al. 2004). This implies that low-income populations with mental illness or SUD are using their limited funds to purchase tobacco in lieu of food or other basic necessities, which impacts not only their health and well-being but also their ability to successfully live in the community.

Smoke is also toxic to others in the environment because secondhand smoke is designated as a known human carcinogen and has immediate adverse effects on the cardiovascular system, contributing to cases of coronary heart disease and lung cancer even in people who do not smoke. There is no risk-free level of exposure to secondhand smoke, and eliminating smoking in indoor spaces is the only way to fully protect others from exposure to it. The U.S. Office of Housing and Urban Development issued a national ruling for smoke-free public housing that went into effect in July 2018 to protect the health of residents, visitors, and staff. Populations with comorbid behavioral health conditions may struggle to comply with such tobacco-free housing regulations if they are not provided with adequate resources and support.

Several studies have now linked tobacco use with worse mental health or other substance use outcomes. A meta-analysis of 26 studies that assessed mental health symptoms showed that anxiety, depression, and stress significantly decreased in people who quit smoking compared with those who continued to smoke (Taylor et al. 2014). In addition, both psychological quality of life and positive affect significantly increased in those who quit during the same period. Although individuals subjectively report using tobacco to reduce anxiety, abundant human and animal data show the opposite: that anxiety is increased with tobacco or nicotine exposure (Garey et al. 2020; Moylan et al. 2012). Because anxiety is also part of the withdrawal syndrome, it is likely that tobacco users receive a temporary relief from withdrawal that is mistaken for an anxiolytic effect. Individuals with SUDs who continue or initiate smoking have worse abstinence and greater odds of SUD relapse (Prochaska et al. 2004; Weinberger et al. 2017).

Tobacco smoke is a potent inducer of the cytochrome P450 1A2 (CYP1A2) isoenzyme, reducing the serum level and presumed effectiveness of important psychiatric medications. This includes commonly used antipsychotics and antidepressants, such as clozapine, olanzapine, and fluvoxamine (Oliveira et al. 2017). Smoking results in the need for higher medication dosages and the potential for medication toxicity during a quit attempt. The major effect is not due to nicotine but to the inhaled polycyclic aromatic hydrocarbons in smoke. Nicotine is metabolized by a different enzyme (CYP2A6), and it (including nicotine replacement medications) has no effect on other medication levels. A comprehensive list of the interactions of smoking with medication was published by the Smoking Cessation Leadership Center, in conjunction with Rx for Change (Table 5–1).

Considerable evidence now shows that smoking is associated with more suicidal thoughts and behaviors. This was recently demonstrated in a meta-analysis of 63 studies involving more than 8 million participants, which showed people who currently smoked were at higher risk

Table 5–1. Drug interactions with tobacco smoke

Drug/Class	Mechanism of interaction and effects
Pharmacokinetic interactions	
Alprazolam (Xanax)	Conflicting data on significance, but possible ↓ plasma concentrations (up to 50%); ↓ half-life (35%).
Bendamustine (Treanda)	Metabolized by CYP1A2. Manufacturer recommends using with caution in smokers due to likely ↓ bendamustine concentrations, with ↑ concentrations of its two active metabolites.
Caffeine	Metabolism (induction of CYP1A2); ↑ clearance (56%). Caffeine levels likely ↑ after cessation.
Chlorpromazine (Thorazine)	↓ Area under the curve (AUC) (36%) and serum concentrations (24%).
	↓ Sedation and hypotension possible in smokers; smokers may require ↑ dosages.
Clopidogrel (Plavix)	↑ Metabolism (induction of CYP1A2) of clopidogrel to its active metabolite.
	Clopidogrel's effects are enhanced in smokers (≥ 10 cigarettes per day): significant ↑ platelet inhibition, ↓ platelet aggregation; improved clinical outcomes have been shown (smokers' paradox; may be dependent on CYP1A2 genotype); tobacco cessation should still be recommended in at-risk populations needing clopidogrel.
Clozapine (Clozaril)	↑ Metabolism (induction of CYP1A2); ↓ plasma concentrations (18%).
	↑ Levels upon cessation may occur; closely monitor drug levels and reduce dose as required to avoid toxicity.
Erlotinib (Tarceva)	↑ Clearance (24%); ↓ trough serum concentrations (twofold).
Flecainide (Tambocor)	↑ Clearance (61%); ↓ trough serum concentrations (25%). Smokers may need ↑ dosages.

Table 5–1. Drug interactions with tobacco smoke (*continued*)

Drug/Class	Mechanism of interaction and effects
Fluvoxamine (Luvox)	↑ Metabolism (induction of CYP1A2); ↑ clearance (24%); ↓ AUC (31%); ↓ Cmax (32%); ↓ Css (39%).
	Dosage modifications not routinely recommended, but smokers may need ↑ dosages.
Haloperidol (Haldol)	↑ Clearance (44%); ↓ serum concentrations (70%); data are inconsistent, therefore clinical significance is unclear.
Heparin	Mechanism unknown but ↑ clearance and ↓ half-life are observed. Smoking has prothrombotic effects.
	Smokers may need ↑ dosages due to PK and PD interactions.
Insulin, subcutaneous	Possible ↓ insulin absorption secondary to peripheral vasoconstriction; smoking may cause the release of endogenous substances that cause insulin resistance.
	PK and PD interactions likely not clinically significant; smokers may need ↑ dosages.
Irinotecan (Camptosar)	↑ Clearance (18%); ↓ serum concentrations of active metabolite, SN-38 (~40%; via induction of glucuronidation); ↓ systemic exposure resulting in lower hematologic toxicity and may reduce efficacy.
	Smokers may need ↑ dosages.
Methadone	Possible ↑ metabolism (induction of CYP1A2, a minor pathway for methadone).
	Carefully monitor response upon cessation.
Mexiletine (Mexitil)	↑ Clearance (25%; via oxidation and glucuronidation); ↓ half-life (36%).
Nintedanib (OFEV®)	Decreased exposure (21%) in smokers.
	No dose adjustment recommended; however, patients should not smoke during use.

Table 5-1. Drug interactions with tobacco smoke (*continued*)

Drug/Class	Mechanism of interaction and effects
Olanzapine (Zyprexa)	↑ Metabolism (induction of CYP1A2); ↑ clearance (98%); ↓ serum concentrations (12%). Dosage modifications are not routinely recommended, but smokers may need ↑ dosages.
Pirfenidone (Esbriet®)	↑ Metabolism (induction of CYP1A2); ↓ AUC (46%) and ↓ Cmax (68%). Decreased exposure in smokers might alter the efficacy profile.
Propranolol (Inderal)	↑ Clearance (77%; via side-chain oxidation and glucuronidation).
Riociguat (Adempas)	↓ Plasma concentrations (by 50%–60%). Smokers may require dosages higher than 2.5 mg three times a day; consider dose reduction upon cessation.
Ropinirole (Requip)	↓ Cmax (30%) and AUC (38%) in a study with patients with restless legs syndrome. Smokers may need ↑ dosages.
Tasimelteon (Hetlioz)	↑ Metabolism (induction of CYP1A2); ↓ drug exposure (40%). Smokers may need ↑ dosages.
Theophylline (Theo-Dur, etc.)	↑ Metabolism (induction of CYP1A2); ↑ clearance (58%–100%); ↓ half-life (63%). Levels should be monitored if smoking is initiated, discontinued, or changed. Maintenance doses are considerably higher in smokers. ↑ Clearance with secondhand smoke exposure.
Tricyclic antidepressants (e.g., imipramine, nortriptyline)	Possible interaction with tricyclic antidepressants in the direction of ↓ blood levels, but the clinical significance is not established.
Tizanidine (Zanaflex)	↓ AUC (30%–40%) and ↓ half-life (10%) observed in male smokers.

Table 5–1. Drug interactions with tobacco smoke (*continued*)

Drug/Class	Mechanism of interaction and effects
Warfarin	↑ Metabolism (induction of CYP1A2) of R-enantiomer; however, S-enantiomer is more potent and effect on INR is inconclusive. Consider monitoring INR upon smoking cessation.

Pharmacodynamic interactions

Benzodiazepines (diazepam, chlordiazepoxide)	↓ Sedation and drowsiness, possibly caused by nicotine stimulation of the central nervous system.
Beta-blockers	Less effective antihypertensive and heart rate control effects, possibly caused by nicotine-mediated sympathetic activation. Smokers may need ↑ dosages.
Corticosteroids, inhaled	**Smokers with asthma may have less of a response to inhaled corticosteroids.**
Hormonal contraceptives	**↑ Risk of cardiovascular adverse effects (e.g., stroke, myocardial infarction, thromboembolism) in women who smoke and use oral contraceptives. Ortho Evra patch users shown to have a twofold ↑ risk of venous thromboembolism compared to oral contraceptive users, likely due to ↑ estrogen exposure (60% higher levels).**
	↑ Risk with age and with heavy smoking (≥15 cigarettes per day) and is quite marked in women ≥35 years old.
Serotonin 5-HT$_1$ receptor agonists (triptans)	This class of drugs may cause coronary vasospasm; caution for use in smokers due to possible unrecognized coronary artery disease.

Note. Many interactions between tobacco smoke and medications have been identified. Note that in most cases it is the tobacco smoke—not the nicotine—that causes these interactions. Tobacco smoke interacts with medications by influencing the absorption, distribution, metabolism, or elimination of other substances, potentially causing an altered pharmacological response. Because of these interactions, people who smoke may require higher dosages of medications. With cessation of smoking, dosage reductions might be needed. Medications with the most clinically significant interactions are in bold font.

Source. Data adapted and updated from Zevin and Benowitz 1999 and Kroon 2007. Table reprinted with permission from Rx for Change: Clinician-Assisted Tobacco Cessation. Copyright © 1999–2025, The Regents of the University of California. All rights reserved.

for suicidal ideation, plan, attempt, and death (Poorolajal and Darvishi 2016). Another meta-analysis found higher rates of completed suicides among those who smoked (Li et al. 2012), and the strongest association may be among people with serious mental illness who smoke (Sankaranarayanan et al. 2015). Although this association does not prove causation, possible theories link biological factors as well as other variables associated with high-risk behaviors and behavioral health comorbidity (Swann et al. 2021). Interestingly, in population-matched analyses, cigarette excise taxes and smoke-free air policies exhibited protective associations with suicide (Grucza et al. 2014).

There is stigma in being someone who smokes, and the social unacceptability of smoking has led to increased perceptions of this. Stigma adds to the burden carried by individuals with SUD, who experience worsening shame and isolation that may reduce their access to care. Within the tobacco control literature, some evidence indicates that self-stigma leads to reductions in smoking, which leads to concerns that this could further marginalize those remaining individuals who continue to smoke and who may be more disadvantaged, with fewer resources available to them to quit.

Case Example

Jean is a 43-year-old with a history of schizophrenia. Their medical history is significant for an irregular heartbeat and high cholesterol. They have a healthy body weight (BMI 23) and smoke about 15 cigarettes per day. About 5 years ago, they underwent a cardiac catheterization and stent placement into one of their coronary arteries. Their mental status has been stable for several years. At mental health visits, they have good eye contact, clear speech, and no obvious hallucinations, paranoia, or delusional thoughts. Their mood is good, and they deny hopelessness or depression. They receive a monthly shot of antipsychotic medication. Jean lives alone but works part time for a brother in a landscaping business, and they enjoy attending church and singing in the choir. Review of the medical record and treatment plan indicate that they are regularly counseled on the risks and benefits of taking antipsychotic medication for schizophrenia. They are advised to use precautions when they are in the sun because their medication increases heat sensitivity. During clinic visits they are advised to eat healthy food, drink adequate water, and include fiber in their daily diet. No mention of tobacco or nicotine appears in the progress notes, the problem list, or the treatment plan.

What Are the Concerns in This Case?

Jean shows evidence of moderate to severe cardiovascular disease for their age, and smoking is a primary risk factor for myocardial infarction, stroke, or other cardiovascular complications. They are at high risk for premature mortality and worsening cardiovascular disease. Perhaps the patient is not aware of this significant risk. Every clinic visit presents an opportunity to educate them about the impact of tobacco on health. Even brief counseling can be helpful in reinforcing this critical message. Perhaps Jean does not want to immediately stop using tobacco, but this cannot be determined from the case described because there is no documentation of them being asked. Many tobacco users are ambivalent about their use and have concerns or fears that keep them from trying to quit, although they recognize it as a problem. Counseling that uses an engaging, motivational approach can explore their wishes and doubts. Sometimes, health care professionals feel uneasy addressing tobacco out of fear that it will upset the patient, but rarely does someone become angry when questioned about tobacco in a caring way. Mental health professionals have more opportunities to intervene with patients like this who are seen frequently. They may also possess additional counseling skills that make them well-suited to provide tobacco intervention. Hearing a consistent message from all health care providers strengthens the message. It is always correct to ask about tobacco and to perform a brief assessment that includes patterns of use, level of dependence, and attitudes about quitting. Providing patients with even brief personalized feedback about tobacco's impact can convey messages of caring and concern. Counseling about the risks of ongoing tobacco use in this patient is as important, or more important, than counseling about antipsychotic medication side effects or diet. Interestingly, these other interventions are provided routinely, without regard for whether the patient is motivated to change their diet, for example. Providing tobacco interventions only for motivated populations misses a sizable group of tobacco users and puts them at risk for worse outcomes including death.

Key Points

- Important disparities in cigarette smoking persist. Some of the highest rates of smoking are found in people who report having a mental illness or another substance use disorder; these rates are at least double those seen in people without these disorders and are worsened by factors such as poverty.

- Some studies have estimated that individuals with current mental illness or substance use disorder make up at least one-third of people in the United States who currently smoke, and they purchase at least one-third of all tobacco products.

- Although tobacco use rates are high in nearly every diagnostic subgroup, it may be more helpful to consider the processes, such as anhedonia, anxiety sensitivity, and distress tolerance, that underlie and contribute to many mental illnesses.

- Biological, psychological, and social factors likely all contribute to higher tobacco use rates and reduced success in quitting among behavioral health populations.

- Using substances to reduce distress or negative affect is a major motivator of substance use and relapse.

- Tobacco contributes to significant health consequences, including the premature loss of life in people with behavioral health conditions, and has a negative impact on other aspects of recovery. Its use is associated with worse mental health illness severity and more relapse back to alcohol and other substances.

References

American Psychiatric Association: Diagnostic and Statistical Manual of Mental Disorders, 5th Edition, Text Revision. Washington, DC, American Psychiatric Association, 2022

Anthenelli RM, Benowitz NL, West R, et al: Neuropsychiatric safety and efficacy of varenicline, bupropion, and nicotine patch in smokers with and without psychiatric disorders (EAGLES): a double-blind, randomised, placebo-controlled clinical trial. Lancet 387(10037):2507–2520, 2016 27116918

Apollonio DE, Malone RE: Marketing to the marginalised: tobacco industry targeting of the homeless and mentally ill. Tob Control 14(6):409–415, 2005 16319365

Audrain-McGovern J, Leventhal AM, Strong DR: The role of depression in the uptake and maintenance of cigarette smoking. Int Rev Neurobiol 124:209–243, 2015 26472531

Bandiera FC, Anteneh B, Le T, et al: Tobacco-related mortality among persons with mental health and substance abuse problems. PLoS One 10(3):e0120581, 2015 25807109

Becker TD, Arnold MK, Ro V, et al: Systematic review of electronic cigarette use (vaping) and mental health comorbidity among adolescents and young adults. Nicotine Tob Res 23(3):415–425, 2021 32905589

Berg SA, Sentir AM, Cooley BS, et al: Nicotine is more addictive, not more cognitively therapeutic in a neurodevelopmental model of schizophrenia produced by neonatal ventral hippocampal lesions. Addict Biol 19(6):1020–1031, 2014 23919443

Breslau N, Novak SP, Kessler RC: Psychiatric disorders and stages of smoking. Biol Psychiatry 55(1):69–76, 2004

Callaghan RC, Veldhuizen S, Jeysingh T, et al: Patterns of tobacco-related mortality among individuals diagnosed with schizophrenia, bipolar disorder, or depression. J Psychiatr Res 48(1):102–110, 2014 24139811

Centers for Disease Control and Prevention: Behavioral Risk Factor Surveillance Survey. Atlanta, GA, Centers for Disease Control and Prevention, 2023. Available at: https://www.cdc.gov/brfss/publications/index.htm. Accessed August 1, 2023.

Chambers RA: Adult hippocampal neurogenesis in the pathogenesis of addiction and dual diagnosis disorders. Drug Alcohol Depend 130(1–3):1–12, 2013 23279925

Charach A, Yeung E, Climans T, et al: Childhood attention-deficit/hyperactivity disorder and future substance use disorders: comparative meta-analyses. J Am Acad Child Adolesc Psychiatry 50(1):9–21, 2011 21156266

Cook BL, Wayne GF, Kafali EN, et al: Trends in smoking among adults with mental illness and association between mental health treatment and smoking cessation. JAMA 311(2):172–182, 2014 24399556

Correll CU: Balancing efficacy and safety in treatment with antipsychotics. CNS Spectr 12(10 Suppl 17):12–20, 2007

Cuthbert BN, Insel TR: Toward the future of psychiatric diagnosis: the seven pillars of RDoC. BMC Medicine 11(1):126, 2013

de Leon J, Diaz FJ: A meta-analysis of worldwide studies demonstrates an association between schizophrenia and tobacco smoking behaviors. Schizophr Res 76(2–3):135–157, 2005 15949648

Delnevo CD, Hrywna M, Lewis MJ: Predictors of smoke-free workplaces by employee characteristics: who is left unprotected? Am J Ind Med 46(2):196–202, 2004 15273973

Farrelly MC, Nonnemaker JM, Watson KA: The consequences of high cigarette excise taxes for low-income smokers. PLoS One 7(9):e43838, 2012 22984447

Garey L, Olofsson H, Garza T, et al: The role of anxiety in smoking onset, severity, and cessation-related outcomes: a review of recent literature. Curr Psychiatry Rep 22(8):38, 2020 32506166

Glasheen C, Hedden SL, Forman-Hoffman VL, et al: Cigarette smoking behaviors among adults with serious mental illness in a nationally representative sample. Ann Epidemiol 24(10):776–780, 2014 25169683

Goodwin RD, Pacek LR, Copeland J, et al: Trends in daily cannabis use among cigarette smokers: United States, 2002–2014. Am J Public Health 108(1):137–142, 2018 29161058

Grant BF, Hasin DS, Chou SP, et al: Nicotine dependence and psychiatric disorders in the United States: results from the National Epidemiologic Survey on Alcohol and Related Conditions. Arch Gen Psychiatry 61(11):1107–1115, 2004 15520358

Gray KM, Upadhyaya HP: Tobacco smoking in individuals with attention-deficit hyperactivity disorder: epidemiology and pharmacological approaches to cessation. CNS Drugs 23(8):661–668, 2009 19594195

Grucza RA, Plunk AD, Krauss MJ, et al: Probing the smoking-suicide association: do smoking policy interventions affect suicide risk? Nicotine Tob Res 16(11):1487–1494, 2014 25031313

Guydish J, Passalacqua E, Pagano A, et al: An international systematic review of smoking prevalence in addiction treatment. Addiction 111(2):220–230, 2016 26392127

Hagman BT, Delnevo CD, Hrywna M, et al: Tobacco use among those with serious psychological distress: results from the National Survey of Drug Use and Health, 2002. Addict Behav 33(4):582–592, 2008 18158218

Han B, Volkow ND, Blanco C, et al: Trends in prevalence of cigarette smoking among US adults with major depression or substance use disorders, 2006–2019. JAMA 327(16):1566–1576, 2022 35471512

Houle B, Siegel M: Smoker-free workplace policies: developing a model of public health consequences of workplace policies barring employment to smokers. Tob Control 18(1):64–69, 2009 19168490

Hunt JJ, Cupertino AP, Gajewski BJ, et al: Staff commitment to providing tobacco dependence in drug treatment: reliability, validity, and results of a national survey. Psychol Addict Behav 28(2):389–395, 2014 24128292

Hurt RD, Offord KP, Croghan IT, et al: Mortality following inpatient addictions treatment: role of tobacco use in a community-based cohort. JAMA 275(14):1097–1103, 1996 8601929

Jamal A, Phillips E, Gentzke AS, et al: Current cigarette smoking among adults—United States, 2016. MMWR Morb Mortal Wkly Rep 67(2):53–59, 2018 29346338

Kassel JD, Stroud LR, Paronis CA: Smoking, stress, and negative affect: correlation, causation, and context across stages of smoking. Psychol Bull 129(2):270–304, 2003 12696841

Kessler RC, Andrews G, Colpe LJ, et al: Short screening scales to monitor population prevalences and trends in non-specific psychological distress. Psychol Med 32(6):959–976, 2002 12214795

Kroon LA: Drug interactions with smoking. Am J Health Syst Pharm 64(18):1917–1921, 2007 17823102

Lawrence D, Mitrou F, Zubrick SR: Smoking and mental illness: results from population surveys in Australia and the United States. BMC Public Health 9:285, 2009 19664203

Lemieux A, al'Absi M: Stress psychobiology in the context of addiction medicine: from drugs of abuse to behavioral addictions, in Progress in Brain Research, Vol 223. Edited by Ekhtiari H, Paulus M. New York, Elsevier, 2016, pp 43–62

Leventhal AM, Zvolensky MJ: Anxiety, depression, and cigarette smoking: a transdiagnostic vulnerability framework to understanding emotion-smoking comorbidity. Psychol Bull 141(1):176–212, 2015 25365764

Li D, Yang X, Ge Z, et al: Cigarette smoking and risk of completed suicide: a meta-analysis of prospective cohort studies. J Psychiatr Res 46(10):1257–1266, 2012 22889465

Mitchell JT, Howard AL, Belendiuk KA, et al: Cigarette smoking progression among young adults diagnosed with ADHD in childhood: a 16-year longitudinal study of children with and without ADHD. Nicotine Tob Res 21(5):638–647, 2019 29538764

Moylan S, Jacka FN, Pasco JA, et al: Cigarette smoking, nicotine dependence and anxiety disorders: a systematic review of population-based, epidemiological studies. BMC Med 10:123, 2012 23083451

Nagawa CS, Wang B, Davis M, et al: Examining pathways between family or peer factors and smoking cessation in a nationally representative US sample of adults with mental health conditions who smoke: a structural equation analysis. BMC Public Health 22(1):1566, 2022 35978318

National Center for Health Statistics: National Health Interview Survey. Atlanta, GA, Centers for Disease Control and Prevention, 2017

Odani S, Agaku IT, Graffunder CM, et al: Tobacco product use among military veterans—United States, 2010–2015. MMWR Morb Mortal Wkly Rep 67(1):7–12, 2018 29324732

Office of the Surgeon General: Smoking Cessation: A Report of the Surgeon General. Washington, DC, U.S. Department of Health and Human Services, 2020. Available at: https://www.ncbi.nlm.nih.gov/books/NBK555591. Accessed August 1, 2023. .

Oliveira P, Ribeiro J, Donato H, et al: Smoking and antidepressants pharmacokinetics: a systematic review. Ann Gen Psychiatry 16:17, 2017 28286537

Parker MA, Cordoba-Grueso WS, Streck JM, et al: Intersectionality of serious psychological distress, cigarette smoking, and substance use disorders in the United States: 2008–2018. Drug Alcohol Depend 228:109095, 2021 34601273

Piper ME, Cook JW, Schlam TR, et al: Anxiety diagnoses in smokers seeking cessation treatment: relations with tobacco dependence, withdrawal, outcome and response to treatment. Addiction 106(2):418–427, 2011 20973856

Poorolajal J, Darvishi N: Smoking and suicide: a meta-analysis. PLoS One 11(7):e0156348, 2016 27391330

Pratt LA, Brody DJ: Depression and smoking in the U.S. household population aged 20 and over, 2005–2008. NCHS Data Brief 34:1–8, 2010

Prochaska JJ, Delucchi K, Hall SM: A meta-analysis of smoking cessation interventions with individuals in substance abuse treatment or recovery. J Consult Clin Psychol 72(6):1144–1156, 2004 15612860

Prochaska JJ, Hall SM, Bero LA: Tobacco use among individuals with schizophrenia: what role has the tobacco industry played? Schizophr Bull 34(3):555–567, 2008 17984298

Rogers E, Sherman S: Tobacco use screening and treatment by outpatient psychiatrists before and after release of the American Psychiatric Association treatment guidelines for nicotine dependence. Am J Public Health 104(1):90–95, 2014 24228666

Sankaranarayanan A, Mancuso S, Wilding H, et al: Smoking, suicidality and psychosis: a systematic meta-analysis. PLoS One 10(9):e0138147, 2015 26372218

Sheffer CE, Williams JM, Erwin DO, et al: Tobacco-related disparities viewed through the lens of intersectionality. Nicotine Tob Res 24(2):285–288, 2022 34555170

Siru R, Hulse GK, Tait RJ: Assessing motivation to quit smoking in people with mental illness: a review. Addiction 104(5):719–733, 2009 19413788

Smith PH, Homish GG, Giovino GA, et al: Cigarette smoking and mental illness: a study of nicotine withdrawal. Am J Public Health 104(2):e127–e133, 2014a 24328637

Smith PH, Mazure CM, McKee SA: Smoking and mental illness in the U.S. population. Tob Control 23(e2):e147–e153, 2014b 24727731

Steinberg ML, Williams JM, Ziedonis DM: Financial implications of cigarette smoking among individuals with schizophrenia. Tob Control 13(2):206, 2004 15175544

Stolz PA, Wehring HJ, Liu F, et al: Effects of cigarette smoking and clozapine treatment on 20-year all-cause and cardiovascular mortality in schizophrenia. Psychiatr Q 90(2):351–359, 2019 30632082

Streck JM, Weinberger AH, Pacek LR, et al: Cigarette smoking quit rates among persons with serious psychological distress in the United States from 2008 to 2016: are mental health disparities in cigarette use increasing? Nicotine Tob Res 22(1):130–134, 2020 30351429

Swann AC, Graham DP, Wilkinson AV, et al: Nicotine inhalation and suicide: clinical correlates and behavioral mechanisms. Am J Addict 30(4):316–329, 2021 34109688

Tam J, Warner KE, Meza R: Smoking and the reduced life expectancy of individuals with serious mental illness. Am J Prev Med 51(6):958–966, 2016 27522471

Taylor G, McNeill A, Girling A, et al: Change in mental health after smoking cessation: systematic review and meta-analysis. BMJ 348:g1151, 2014 24524926

Trainor K, Leavey G: Barriers and facilitators to smoking cessation among people with severe mental illness: a critical appraisal of qualitative studies. Nicotine Tob Res 19(1):14–23, 2017 27613905

U.S. Department of Health and Human Services: Preventing Tobacco Use Among Youth and Young Adults: A Report of the Surgeon General. Atlanta, GA, U.S. Department of Health and Human Services, Centers for Disease Control and Prevention, National Center for Chronic Disease Prevention and Health Promotion, Office on Smoking and Health, 2012

Veldhuizen S, Callaghan RC: Cause-specific mortality among people previously hospitalized with opioid-related conditions: a retrospective cohort study. Ann Epidemiol 24(8):620–624, 2014 25084705

Weinberger AH, Desai RA, McKee SA: Nicotine withdrawal in U.S. smokers with current mood, anxiety, alcohol use, and substance use disorders. Drug Alcohol Depend 108(1–2):7–12, 2010 20006451

Weinberger AH, Platt J, Esan H, et al: Cigarette smoking is associated with increased risk of substance use disorder relapse: a nationally representative, prospective longitudinal investigation. J Clin Psychiatry 78(2):e152–e160, 2017 28234432

Weinberger AH, Chaiton MO, Zhu J, et al: Trends in the prevalence of current, daily, and nondaily cigarette smoking and quit ratios by depression status in the U.S.: 2005–2017. Am J Prev Med 58(5):691–698, 2020 32156490

Young WJ, Delnevo CD, Singh B, et al: Tobacco treatment knowledge and practices among US psychiatrists. Community Ment Health J 59(1):185–191, 2023 35768703

Zevin S, Benowitz NL: Drug interactions with tobacco smoking: an update. Clinical Pharmacokinetics 36(6):425–438, 1999 10427467

6

Behavioral Interventions for Individuals Who Are Ready to Quit Smoking

Most of the public health interventions for smoking are primarily designed to motivate people to attempt to quit smoking. These interventions include mass media and other education campaigns on the harms to health from smoking and from environmental tobacco smoke; increases in the price of cigarettes via taxation; and implementation of smoke-free air policies in work and other public places (primarily to prevent exposure to environmental tobacco smoke and make it far more inconvenient to continue to smoke). The effect of such interventions is to shift the whole population along the stages of change from precontemplation to contemplation of quitting, preparing to quit, and actually making a quit attempt.

Partly as a result of these public health interventions, the proportion of people who smoke and attempt to quit each year was consistently above 50% in the United States from 2009 to 2018 (Creamer et al. 2019). Successful smoking cessation per year increased from 6.3% in 2009 to 7.5% in 2018 (calculated as the proportion of people who recently smoked cigarettes and have quit for at least 6 months during the past year). This resulted in an increase in the "lifetime quit ratio" (the percentage of people who ever smoked cigarettes and have currently quit smoking) from 52% in 2009 to 62% in 2018. However, because many of these people finally succeeded in quitting smoking in their late middle-age or older, after they had already developed smoking-caused diseases, there is enormous room for improvement in the smoking cessation rate (and resulting health benefits) by providing people who smoke with effective evidence-based treatment earlier in their life and continuing to provide treatment until they successfully quit.

During 2018–2019, 77% of people in the United States who smoked expressed a desire to quit smoking. Among the 51% who had made a past-year quit attempt during that time, only 34% reported using some type of evidence-based smoking cessation treatment, including an FDA-approved nicotine replacement therapy (NRT; 24.7%) or prescription medication (12.1%), telephone quitline (3.6%), in-person one-on-one counseling (5.2%), class or group counseling (2.1%), digital Web or smartphone application (2.6%), or medication and counseling combination treatment (6.1%) (Leventhal et al. 2022). Because the vast majority of quit attempts are "unaided," a large proportion of successful attempts also are unaided, leading some to claim that because most people quit smoking on their own, there is no need for treatment. However, very good data show that the average 40-year-old person who started smoking in their teens already will have made more than 20 unsuccessful quit attempts in the interim (Borland et al. 2012).

In this chapter, we describe the evidence for behavioral treatments for people who are ready to try to quit smoking and summarize the typical formats used to provide those effective treatments.

Summary of Evidence of Efficacy of Various Behavioral Treatments

Clear evidence demonstrates that brief advice (lasting <15 minutes) can improve quit rates and largely increase quit attempts and that more intensive individual and group counseling can provide higher quit rates. All of these proven counseling modalities tend to produce higher quit rates when added to pharmacotherapy than either counseling or pharmacotherapy alone.

The risk ratios shown in Table 6–1 reflect the proportional increase in long-term (≥6 months) abstinence rates when the intervention is compared with minimal intervention or usual care. These effect estimates are based on meta-analyses of randomized controlled trials. The absolute quit rates cannot easily be compared across treatments because the characteristics of the trial participants in the different trials may vary. For example, trials of brief physician advice typically

Table 6–1. Efficacy of behavioral methods

Method (trials, *N*)	Compared with minimal or usual care unless otherwise noted, *RR (95% CI)*
Behavioral counseling	
Individual counseling (17)	1.57 (1.40–1.77)
Group counseling (13)	1.88 (1.52–2.33)
Telephone quitline counseling (13)	1.38 (1.19–1.61)
Clinician counseling	
Brief advice (17)	1.66 (1.42–1.94)
Brief counseling (11)	1.86 (1.60–2.15)
Brief counseling (vs. brief advice)	1.37 (1.20–1.56)
Counseling added to pharmacotherapy (65)	1.15 (1.08–1.22) vs. pharmacotherapy alone

Source.   Adapted from Rigotti et al. 2022.

include all people who smoke, regardless of their interest in quitting or dependence, and improve the long-term quit rate from 4.8% to 8.0%. Slightly more intensive counseling by trained nonphysician counselors can increase the long-term quit rate from 7.7% to 11.4%, and in these trials, the participants who smoke may have more interest in quitting and greater dependence (which is why they consented to a study of counseling for smoking cessation).

Overall, it appears that most behavioral interventions that encourage a structured quit attempt and provide encouragement to persist with quit attempt are likely to be helpful. Relatively intensive in-person interventions appear to result in the highest short-term quit rates (e.g., at 1- to 3-month follow-ups), but they also require relatively high motivation and time commitment on the part of patients and thus can be more difficult to implement in a manner that has "reach," in the sense of being able to help a large number of people in the local target community to quit smoking.

Given that abstinence rates are improved by the offer of effective smoking-cessation medicines, as discussed in previous chapters, and that counseling plus medication is consistently supported as the most effective treatment format, over the rest of this chapter we describe in more detail typical formats used in each of these behavioral treatments.

Brief Individual Advice (Advise)

Brief advice can be performed by any health professional and can be as brief as 30 seconds or as long as 10 minutes if further assessment or medication advice is included. In the context of the "5A's" (Ask, Advise, Assess, Assist, Arrange Follow-Up), this composes the "Advise" component. One example of a brief, simple piece of advice that can be provided after identifying that a patient currently smokes tobacco (Foulds et al. 2010) would be to say something such as,

> "As your clinician, I want you to know that the single best thing you can do for your health right now is to quit smoking. Every year that you continue smoking likely reduces your healthy life span by around 3 months. I understand that it may not be an easy thing to do, but there are now treatments that have been shown to be effective, and I am familiar with those treatments and can help provide them. I believe it is very important for your health that we get started on this."

When this type of accurate but encouraging advice is followed up with a question about the patient's interest in quitting, it is more likely to receive a positive response, which can lead directly to a more detailed assessment and discussion about treatment options. If the clinician is unlikely to have any further contact with the patient in the near future (e.g., in the emergency department or an urgent care center), then the next step that might be taken, very briefly, is to explain the benefits of obtaining telephone counseling and refer the person directly to the free national quitline (1-800-QUIT-NOW).

Brief Individual Counseling (Assist)

The key components of providing brief counseling that go beyond brief advice are to briefly assess dependence and motivation, provide information on pharmacotherapy options, arrange a target quit date, and arrange a follow-up (either in person or by telephone) around 1 week later (and certainly within 1 month) to assess progress, check appropriate medication use, and encourage continued effort to remain abstinent. Ideally, the individual providing brief smoking cessation counseling should have access to a portable exhaled carbon monoxide (eCO) monitor, so that eCO can be measured at baseline while the patient is still smoking and again at the follow-up. The patient should be informed that this will be measured at follow-up and that if they have quit, their eCO should be significantly lower. This provides additional motivation to attend the follow-up and to be abstinent. Here is an example script, adapted from a study of smoking cessation treatment (Foulds et al. 2015):

> "Your exhaled carbon monoxide reading was 20. This is much higher than that of a nonsmoker (typically 0–4). It means that the carbon monoxide, or CO, from inhaled cigarette smoking is binding to the red blood cells that carry oxygen in your blood and displacing oxygen. This means that your heart has to do more work to supply oxygen to your body, and it is part of the reason why smoking causes serious cardiovascular diseases such as heart attack or a stroke. It is very important to get that number down. The good news is that when you stop smoking, the concentration of CO in your body will return to that of a never-smoker within a week. So it is really important that you attend the next appointment, use the nicotine patches, and succeed in stopping smoking. We will measure your CO levels at the next appointment, and you will be able to see the improvement when you quit smoking."

Intensive Individual Counseling

Whereas in many areas of behavioral treatment, "intensive" typically refers to many individual appointments, at least weekly, lasting at least 1 hour and continuing for months, in the field of smoking cessation, intensive counseling typically includes any counseling that lasts for more than 15 minutes on more than two occasions. In tobacco dependence treatment, a typical format would involve an assessment appointment lasting 40–60 minutes, a follow-up on or near the target quit date, and then weekly appointments lasting until 1 month after the target quit date. If resources permit, additional, less frequent follow-up appointments may be offered to provide ongoing support and help prevent relapse, and a final follow-up visit is arranged at 6 months for evaluation purposes and to advise on tapering off any continuing medication use. It is considered good practice to "front-load" appointments during the first month because this is the time when nicotine withdrawal symptoms are most prominent and when the patient may need regular advice on medication use and other behavior changes to help maintain abstinence. People often have the occasional "slip" (smoking an isolated cigarette) or "lapse" (smoking one cigarette, immediately followed by further smoking over the next few days). It can be helpful to discuss how these slips happened and what changes can be made to ensure they do not happen again (e.g., did the patient get rid of all their cigarettes, go into a predictably high-risk situation without being prepared, use another psychoactive substance that impaired their judgment?). Once the patient has achieved 3 weeks or longer without smoking, they will typically start to find that abstinence is becoming easier and that their urges to smoke are becoming noticeably less severe and less frequent. This gives them more confidence that they can succeed. Part of counseling involves reminding patients how much effort they have put in to achieving a period of abstinence and encouraging them to continue the behaviors that have helped them succeed. The evidence suggests that there is a dose-response effect related to the number of counseling sessions received from a trained counselor (at least four or five sessions), and that either varenicline or combination NRT (typically the nicotine patch plus a short-acting product such as nicotine gum, lozenge, nasal spray, or inhaler) has the best outcomes (Rigotti et al. 2022).

Group Counseling

Group smoking cessation counseling appears to be at least as effective as individual counseling and has the advantage of being able to treat a much larger number of people in the same time it would take to treat a single patient with individual counseling. A review by Kotsen et al. (2019) included data from 11 observational studies (i.e., not randomized trials) comparing the outcome of group versus individual treatment. In all trials, group treatment had higher 4-week CO-validated quit rates (range 36%–67%) than individual treatment at the same site (range 19%–53%). This review concluded that the best-practice group treatments for tobacco dependence are generalizable from research to clinical settings and are feasible in various settings with good results.

Many of the studies included in the review were based in either the United Kingdom national smoking cessation services or the New Jersey "quit centers." Treatment providers in both settings were trained and encouraged to use a specific format of group treatment, originally described as "withdrawal-oriented group treatment for smokers" (Hajek 1994a). Pharmacotherapy is a cornerstone of this type of group treatment, and because the rationale and evidence for using approved medications to reduce nicotine withdrawal and cravings is explained in detail in Chapter 7, here we discuss the behavioral and practical aspects of withdrawal-oriented group treatment.

Group support is used to help people maintain the willpower necessary to get through the difficult first few weeks, when craving and withdrawal are at their worst. The group meets once per week for 6 consecutive weeks on the same day of the week, with the first group meeting being the "preparation" meeting and the second meeting being on the "quit day." By the last group meeting, most of the participants will have come through the 2- to 4-week withdrawal phase together. To encourage group support, the therapist should behave in a manner that facilitates interaction and discussion among group members, rather than behaving like a teacher, with the group members all sitting quietly and listening for advice (as is more common in traditional groups). The therapist obviously must provide some structure and information (e.g., on the use of medications, withdrawal), but evidence has demonstrated that "group-oriented" (rather than "therapist-oriented") groups do better at stopping smoking (Hajek 1994b). Certain techniques can be used to foster group support and communication, and these are described in more detail in the "Procedures at Each Group Meeting" section.

The available evidence suggests that more-intensive treatments are more effective than less-intensive treatments. However, services must be mindful that prospective patients will have busy lives and that the greater the number of attendances required, the lower the number of prospective patients who will be able to make a commitment to attend. The evidence also suggests a "law of diminishing returns" as the intensity and complexity of treatments being provided increase. Thus, it cannot be assumed that a five-session treatment will result in 20% more successes than a four-session treatment. One final point to consider is the cost and time efficiency of the treatment being offered. Group treatments have a significant advantage over individual treatment in this regard. The group format we present here has been developed over a number of years with these considerations in mind.

Assessment and Preparation of Patients

Who Is Suitable?

Ideally, all potential patients should be seen individually for an assessment prior to being included in the group. This interview can establish whether the person is motivated to stop smoking, understands the treatment being offered, and is keen to participate. Each patient's eCO level should be measured and explained during this assessment. The following list gives an idea of positive and negative indications for the treatment being described here.

Positive indications
- Has a strong desire to stop smoking completely
- Smokes daily and has had some prior difficulty quitting
- Is willing to use medication for at least 4 weeks
- Is able to commit time to attend six group meetings

Negative indications
- Is unsure about intention to stop smoking now
- Is very socially anxious
- Has behavioral characteristics that may be unhelpful in a group context (e.g., unstable mental health problems, unstable drug/ alcohol abuse)

The treatment has been shown to achieve a success rate of about one-half to two-thirds—that is, if 15 people attended the "quit day" group meeting, one could expect that approximately 8–10 members would be abstinent at the sixth group meeting 1 month later (Foulds et al. 2015). The type of participants recruited will largely determine the actual success rate achieved in any one group. The added treatment effect provided in a group setting partly comes from the effect of seeing others succeed and being motivated to keep up with them. The therapist should therefore resist the temptation to include "doubtful" participants in the group because this can lead to a negative group effect that comes from seeing others fail or not even try very hard to succeed. Potential participants who are not thought to be suitable for the group can be offered treatment or counseling on an individual basis, which has been shown to produce good success rates (Foulds et al. 2006).

Once a person is deemed suitable for group inclusion, they then should be given a clear idea of what to expect from the group. They should be informed about the number and timing of meetings and told that they will be expected to quit completely beginning the day of the second meeting. They should also be informed that the success rate from similar groups at the end of treatment is about 50% (i.e., at the last meeting, 50% of participants report not having taken a single puff during the previous 7 days, validated by their eCO levels) (Foulds et al. 2015). The target group size at the first meeting should be about 16–18 people. One can usually expect about a 25% dropout from the number booked for the first meeting. Starting with at least 10 people in the group also ensures that by the final group meeting there are participants who have succeeded in quitting and therefore ensures there is a "feel-good factor" for staff and participants alike.

Procedures at Each Group Meeting

Basic recordkeeping should be carried out at the start of each group, with attendance, self-reported cigarettes smoked in the previous week, self-reported treatment medication use, and eCO being recorded for each participant as they arrive each week. They should also be given the opportunity to discuss more personal issues briefly at the end of the group meetings or in separate sessions or telephone calls.

Group 1

The first meeting is obviously important because it sets the tone for following meetings. The ethos to be encouraged is one of determination to quit completely, with members supporting each other's efforts and gaining from each other's experiences. However, the idea is to establish expectations of success and to *not* dwell too much on the difficulties or support excuses or "cutting down." Group cohesion should be encouraged by arranging the seats in a circle. Every participant should be given a folded card and asked to write their first name in large letters on the front and to place it in front of them. The therapist welcomes everyone and gives a brief introduction and then suggests that everyone briefly introduce themselves, sharing their name, some piece of information about themself (e.g., a hobby), and perhaps the reason they want to stop smoking. A volunteer should start this process, and then it should proceed around the circle.

After introductions, the therapist should remind participants of the reason they are there—to stop smoking completely from the quit day onward—and ask if anyone is unclear about this. This topic usually starts off some discussion because typically at least one member is unsure of their ability to stop "cold turkey" or the wisdom of doing so. This concern can lead naturally to the therapist introducing medication, explaining the rationale for its use, and explaining clearly how it should be used. Some time may need to be spent clarifying expectations about medication and discussing the practicalities of its use. When patients are using prescription-only medications, it may be helpful to have a physician, physician assistant, or advanced practice nurse in attendance for the first two group meetings to discuss the medications and to monitor side effects. In addition to those who have failed to quit cold turkey, even more members likely have failed repeatedly to cut down. The group should be encouraged to spend the week before their quit date preparing for it, thinking about the things that caused them to relapse during previous quit attempts, and making a plan for how to deal with those types of situations. Participants should be encouraged to discuss difficult situations and to seek advice from the group on how to cope.

Therapists leading the group should avoid making speeches but instead encourage group members to give their views. Whenever the group is engaging in constructive discussion, the therapist should resist the temptation to intervene with their "expert" opinion. Indeed, whenever possible, questions directed at the therapist should be redirected back to the group, with the therapist only intervening to correct inaccurate information or to keep everyone focused on the goal at hand. The therapist may discourage conversation being directed to them specifically by intentionally not returning the member's eye contact when being addressed. Co-facilitation by two therapists is recommended to speed up data collection at the start of the group meeting and to reduce the extent that the group feels as though a single individual is leading them.

A useful ritual for the end of each group meeting is to ask for volunteers to stand up and make a promise to the group that they will not smoke another cigarette between the current day and the next meeting. Every participant should be encouraged to follow this procedure and to publicly commit that they will attend the group next week. Sometimes patients will have a valid reason why they cannot attend the next meeting. They should make a commitment to call the therapist before the session to say how they are doing so that it can be shared with the group. Others may be reluctant to make such a promise, and this is allowable, but anyone refusing to throw away their cigarettes should be questioned thoroughly and basically be challenged about this. Asking the group whether they think it is a good idea to keep any remaining tobacco handy can easily accomplish this. Another way for the member and the group to consider this issue is for the therapist to ask them, "Would you buy a big chocolate cake and put it in the fridge the day before you planned to start a weight loss diet?"

Group meetings should last at least 50 minutes; 90 minutes is preferable. Any remaining time may be spent discussing issues such as how to avoid high-risk situations, change old habits, and so on. Because every group member will be encouraged to speak at least briefly at the beginning (introductions) and end (commitments) of every meeting, plus have the opportunity to speak during the meeting, 50 minutes may be too tight for a group of 15, and even 90 minutes can feel rushed when the group starts with more than 20 participants. Meetings should finish with a reminder about next week's meeting time and the expectation of seeing everyone at that time as "nonsmokers."

Group 2 (Quit Day)

Group 2 follows a similar format. All patients should be seen individually prior to the start of the meeting to record their eCO level, number of cigarettes smoked today (or in the past week at future meetings), and medication use. Patients are typically very pleased to see that their eCO concentration has dropped significantly within the first day of stopping smoking. Patients should again place their name card in front of their chair. The therapist begins by going around the group in a circle asking each member to report how they fared since the previous meeting (i.e., how many cigarettes they smoked, what medication they used, what has been difficult, and what has helped). All successes (e.g., no tobacco so far since the first day) should be enthusiastically praised, and some spontaneous applause may be appropriate. The group should be encouraged to give advice from their own experience to members who are having difficulties and to not accept uncritically any excuses that indicate that someone is not prioritizing their quit attempt.

This is a good opportunity to ask about withdrawal symptoms and to impart information about their duration, severity, and any other concerns. This may be a good time to point out that some people's difficulties are partly caused by them not using enough of their NRT, because most people do not use the recommended amount. Participants should be encouraged to use their NRT in the group and to get into the habit of regular NRT use.

The other main issue that may be discussed at this meeting is that of dealing with friends and family members who smoke and who offer cigarettes and how to deal with these situations. As before, the meeting should finish with everyone promising not to smoke during the coming week and promising to attend the next group meeting tobacco-free.

Groups 3, 4, and 5

The next three meetings follow a similar format, covering slightly different issues each week. For example, at week 3 it may be appropriate to discuss the difficulty of keeping up the enthusiasm and motivation now that the novelty of quitting is beginning to wear off. Participants should be reminded that it is crucial not to be drawn into the idea that "one little cigarette won't do any harm" and that total abstinence is the goal. The group ethos should continue to focus on achieving and maintaining abstinence throughout. Whenever appropriate, cohesion-enhancing games should be organized; for example, the group might start a "buddy" system whereby each member pairs with one or two others, and they exchange contact information with the aim of supporting and encouraging each other throughout the week. This could be combined with a game in which the partners (who should be having roughly equal success in quitting) nominate a cause or charity that is abhorrent to them both, and then agree on an amount of money (e.g., $5) that they will *both* donate to that unworthy cause if *even one* of them smokes during the following week. Such an arrangement should not be confused with gambling, because neither party receives money.

Participants who have a slip or relapse should be strongly encouraged to continue attending meetings to receive support and encouragement as they attempt to abstain again. When such participants do attend group meetings, they should be praised for their courage in attending but firmly encouraged to become abstinent immediately and to keep roughly on track with the rest of the group.

At the end of week 5, all group participants are again asked to promise abstinence. This time, they should be reminded that the next week's session is the last and will partly consist of a celebration, with (nonalcoholic) drinks and snacks included. The celebration will be even better if all participants are able to achieve abstinence during the last week.

Group 6

The final group meeting starts off as usual, with each member reporting their experiences during the previous week. Issues typically discussed at this meeting include dealing with increased appetite and weight gain; when the cravings will go away; future high-risk relapse situations to be wary of (e.g., holidays, high-stress, alcohol-associated situations); and the methods and timing for reducing medication use. Some participants may think it would be helpful to keep in touch with other members for continued support, and this should be encouraged. The meeting may then take on a lighter note, with all successful participants (i.e., those who have not smoked at all during the previous 7 days) being presented with an "I'm a nonsmoker" badge and a certificate, and everyone having soft drinks and party snacks. (People who have just stopped smoking will generally be rather hungry!)

Typical Outcomes From Group Treatment

A clinical trial conducted in central Pennsylvania and published in 2015 that involved 225 people seeking help to quit smoking used the group format just described (Foulds et al. 2015). Group attendance, NRT use, mean eCO level, and CO-confirmed abstinence for at least the past 7 days at each of the six sessions were reported. The 225 participants were assigned to 22 separate groups, with an average starting group size of 10 members (range 5–22). At the last (sixth) group meeting, 116/225 (~52%) attended and reported no smoking in the previous week, validated by an eCO level below 10 parts per million (ppm). Attendance at the previous group session was about 73% (164/225). Attendance among those assessed declined from 88% at group 1 to 53% at the penultimate meeting (group 5), with some nonattendance due to schedule conflicts but more due to having difficulty quitting and dropping out. Attendance at the sixth group meeting increased because it had been emphasized that this was an important meeting to attend and to do so smoking-abstinent. The mean eCO level among those attending the groups decreased from just over 20 ppm at group 1 (still smoking) to 7 ppm at the quit-day session (group 2) and 6 ppm at group 6.

These outcomes are fairly typical for this type of treatment that combines withdrawal-oriented group treatment with individual assessment and strong encouragement to use evidence-based pharmacotherapy. A large-scale evaluation of outcomes in the English smoking cessation service reported 4-week CO-validated outcomes for 4,780 people who participated in group treatment and reported that just over 50% had quit at the 1-month point (corresponding to the last group meeting in this type of closed-group format) (Dobbie et al. 2015). Perhaps the strongest data supporting the efficacy of group-based smoking cessation treatment (combined with pharmacotherapy) came from the U.S. Lung Health Study (Anthonisen et al. 1994), in which almost 6,000 middle-aged participants who smoked and had asymptomatic airway obstruction were randomly assigned to either usual care or intensive group-based smoking cessation treatment combined with nicotine gum. Five years later, 22% of the intervention group had quit within the first year and remained abstinent, compared with 5% of the usual-care control group. At 15-year follow-up, significantly more of the group who had received intensive group-based smoking cessation treatment were still alive (Anthonisen et al. 2005).

Common challenges to running regular group treatment are 1) that it is necessary to recruit enough people who can start group treatment at the same time (target starting group size is >14, anticipating a few initial dropouts and more during the first month); and 2) that some of those who found the group support helpful will request more sessions or think they are at greater risk of relapse when the group sessions end and when it is time to reduce or stop their smoking cessation medication. For these reasons, it is more practical to conduct regular smoking cessation groups in relatively large urban centers rather than in rural areas. Many therapists who attempt to start a smoking cessation group with only three or four people registered for the first meeting become disillusioned when only two show up, and by week 4, the group has dissolved. This situation is not reinforcing for either the therapist or the one person who might still be attending. Starting with at least 14 registered participants almost guarantees that by the last few sessions, at least six or seven people will still be attending and almost all will no longer be smoking.

Another option is to run open groups in addition to the 6-week closed-group format. Some centers use closed groups as their primary treatment modality but then offer "graduates" from the 6-week closed group the option of attending a regular open group that meets on another day or evening, largely for continuing support and relapse prevention. For closed-group formats, only those attending one of the first two sessions can attend the rest of the meetings, and attendance at all six sessions and quitting on the same target quit date are strongly encouraged to ensure participants are all going through the same stages of quitting together at the same time.

Some services have found the closed-group format to be too difficult to organize and prefer to use the same basic format except in an open group. In this format, new participants who join the group are encouraged to follow the same steps on a similar time scale to the 6-week group but can continue to attend for as long as they wish and can drop in at any time when they need the support. These open, rolling groups allow people to join at any time and tend to have a core group of regular attendees who have succeeded in quitting and value the group support to help them avoid relapse. The Dobbie et al. (2015) study based in England found that this style of open-group format achieved a similar CO-validated cigarette abstinence rate at 4 weeks (52%) as the closed-group format.

Telephone "Quitline" Counseling

Every part of the United States, and many other countries, has access to publicly funded evidence-based "quitline" services (Stead et al. 2006). These services are typically run by a relatively large vendor organization, on a competitive contract basis, providing quitline counseling for multiple states and/or employers as well as other specialized subgroups (e.g., veterans or people who speak specific languages). In the United States, each state is responsible for running its own quitline through a national quitline portal (1-800-QUIT-NOW).

These services provide evidence-based training to their counseling staff, use modern computer systems to manage calls, and deliver outbound, proactive callbacks. A fairly typical format entitles each caller to one assessment/registration call and four to six subsequent counseling calls; for the latter, the service will call the person at agreed times to provide encouragement, tips, and support. Many quitline vendors also have specialized counseling protocols for specific groups (e.g., pregnant or teenage callers). Almost all quitline services also provide NRT at no cost, mailed to the caller's home, and some can also provide the prescription medicines bupropion and varenicline.

Over the past decade, U.S. quitlines have managed an annual call volume in the range of 800,000–1,300,000, serving 285,000–446,000 unique tobacco users each year. The great advantage of these services is their ease of access to the public, as well as ease of referral from clinicians. Another advantage is that the vendors have become experts in providing tobacco cessation counseling based on solid evidence. These advantages can also provide challenges because quitlines must be prepared to handle calls from people with a wide range of motivation for quitting, as well as for those desiring participation in the optimal treatment protocol (e.g., a combination of NRT use and participation in at least five counseling calls post registration). Quitlines must be prepared to manage these varying levels of motivation, and their counseling protocols must be flexible enough to help each person according to their level of motivation in each specific call. Another challenge for quitlines is that to provide maximum efficiency they must have a large staff, so each caller does not typically speak to the same counselor on every call.

Over the past decade, quitline services have been at the forefront of integrating telephone smoking cessation services with other technology-based formats, including automated digital messaging and texts, Web chat–based coaching (software designed to simulate conversations with humans), text or internet-based coaching, and mobile phone–based applications. Although some components of these services are solidly supported by evidence from randomized controlled trials (e.g., telephone cessation counseling and smoking-cessation text messaging), others are relatively recent developments and have yet to be fully evaluated.

Conclusion

A common and likely critical element in all behavioral interventions to assist smoking cessation is that they offer a logical plan of action for the person to follow, whether it be a highly structured and directed plan, as in a closed, withdrawal-oriented smoking cessation group, or a plan that is decided by the person during counseling, as in telephone counseling provided by a quitline. The efficacy of these counseling modalities in randomized controlled trials indicates that people benefit from receiving regular reminders about their plan and encouragement to persist with it. Automated text messages delivered to the person's cell phone are an efficient way to provide such prompts, but receiving social support from other people appears to be an important treatment ingredient, whether that social support is provided by a counselor, other people attempting to quit in a group treatment, or simply the support and encouragement of friends or relatives. Finally, although the evidence from clinical trials is critical, no two people are identical, so all people who smoke should be informed about and provided with a range of treatment options. Some may prefer the flexibility of telephone counseling, while others may prefer the regular appointments and social support provided by group treatment.

Case Example

Angelica (age 53) has smoked since she was 17 years old. She has tried to quit more times than she can remember, sometimes by gradually reducing cigarette consumption but usually by just deciding not to smoke on a particular day (e.g., her fiftieth birthday, when cigarette taxes were raised, or on New Year's Day). She has also occasionally purchased nicotine patches and lozenges but has never quit smoking for longer than 2 weeks. She is seeing her family doctor for a prescription for varenicline. Her doctor has suggested that she may benefit from counseling, but Angelica's initial response is that she does not see how talking about this with a stranger will help, and she doesn't have money to pay for it.

What Are the Concerns in This Case?

This case is not unusual in that the patient has concerns about the financial cost of smoking cessation counseling, as well as doubts about whether it will be helpful for her. It may be useful to briefly explain how counseling can assist and that no or low-cost options are available. For example, quitline counselors are trained and have experience in helping people quit smoking. They may help the caller decide on a plan and call back at agreed times, and this service is both free and can help maintain motivation by making the caller accountable to someone else. Finally, strong evidence from controlled clinical trials has shown that engaging in telephone counseling can increase the chances of successfully quitting smoking.

Key Points

- Solid evidence indicates that behavioral support can increase a person's chances of successfully quitting smoking.
- Evidence also consistently reinforces the idea that more support leads to improved quit rates (whether measured by number of sessions, minutes of counseling, or number of support modalities used).
- Growing evidence shows that methods employing modern technologies (e.g., telephone, text messages, internet-based, video calls) also increase quit rates.
- People who smoke should be informed about the behavioral support options that are available and told that there is good evidence that these treatments actually help participants to quit.
- Combining behavioral support with pharmacotherapy typically leads to the best outcomes, but each of these components can also help on its own.

References

Anthonisen NR, Connett JE, Kiley JP, et al: Effects of smoking intervention and the use of an inhaled anticholinergic bronchodilator on the rate of decline of FEV1: the Lung Health Study. JAMA 272(19):1497–1505, 1994 7966841

Anthonisen NR, Skeans MA, Wise RA, et al: The effects of a smoking cessation intervention on 14.5-year mortality: a randomized clinical trial. Ann Intern Med 142(4):233–239, 2005 15710956

Borland R, Partos TR, Yong H-H, et al: How much unsuccessful quitting activity is going on among adult smokers? Data from the International Tobacco Control four country cohort survey. Addiction 107(3):673–682, 2012 21992709

Creamer MR, Wang TW, Babb S, et al: Tobacco product use and cessation indicators among adults—United States, 2018. MMWR Morb Mortal Wkly Rep 68(45):1013–1019, 2019 31725711

Dobbie F, Hiscock R, Leonardi-Bee J, et al: Evaluating Long-term Outcomes of NHS Stop Smoking Services (ELONS): a prospective cohort study. Health Technol Assess 19(95):1–156, 2015 26565129

Foulds J, Gandhi KK, Steinberg MB, et al: Factors associated with quitting smoking at a tobacco dependence treatment clinic. Am J Health Behav 30(4):400–412, 2006 16787130

Foulds J, Schmelzer AC, Steinberg MB: Treating tobacco dependence as a chronic illness and a key modifiable predictor of disease. Int J Clin Pract 64(2):142–146, 2010 19919548

Foulds J, Veldheer S, Hrabovsky S, et al: The effect of motivational lung age feedback on short-term quit rates in smokers seeking intensive group treatment: a randomized controlled pilot study. Drug Alcohol Depend 153:271–277, 2015 26051163

Hajek P: Helping smokers to overcome tobacco withdrawal: background and practice of withdrawal-oriented therapy, in Interventions for Smokers: An International Perspective. Baltimore, MD, Williams & Wilkins, 1994a, pp 29–46

Hajek P: Treatments for smokers. Addiction 89(11):1543–1549, 1994b 7841869

Kotsen C, Santorelli ML, Bloom EL, et al: A narrative review of intensive group tobacco treatment: clinical, research, and US policy recommendations. Nicotine Tob Res 21(12):1580–1589, 2019 30124924

Leventhal AM, Dai H, Higgins ST: Smoking cessation prevalence and inequalities in the United States: 2014–2019. J Natl Cancer Inst 114(3):381–390, 2022 34850047

Rigotti NA, Kruse GR, Livingstone-Banks J, et al: Treatment of tobacco smoking: a review. JAMA 327(6):566–577, 2022 35133411

Stead LF, Perera R, Lancaster T: Telephone counselling for smoking cessation. Cochrane Database Syst Rev 3(3):CD002850, 2006 16855992

7

Pharmacological and Other Biological Treatments for Tobacco Use Disorder

Pharmacological treatments for tobacco use disorder (TUD) have a strong evidence base for increasing the likelihood of a successful quit attempt. These medications reduce tobacco withdrawal symptoms and craving and block the pleasurable effects of nicotine in the brain. They are associated with a 1.5- to 2.5-times increase in quitting success, and although they are most effective when combined with counseling, they are also effective when used alone (U.S. Department of Health and Human Services 2020). Several medications have FDA approval for the treatment of TUD: four types of nicotine replacement therapy (NRTs), bupropion sustained-release (SR), and varenicline. All of these medications have been proven effective compared with placebo across numerous randomized clinical trials. None is associated with a risk for major adverse cardiovascular events (i.e., cardiovascular death, myocardial infarction, or stroke) (Benowitz et al. 2018).

A more aggressive use of pharmacotherapy has become the norm as the evidence base has increased, and nearly every tobacco user can benefit from treatment. Advances include use of the medications for extended periods (i.e., relapse prevention, pretreatment prior to the quit day, reduction-to-quit paradigms) of weeks or longer to help patients reduce smoking successfully and to ultimately quit. Although some of these strategies are technically off-label in the United States, many are clinically useful and consistent with a motivationally oriented approach that tries to engage as many tobacco users as possible into treatment. Here we review basic as well as advanced topics in the use of pharmacological treatments for TUD.

Current evidence supports two treatments with better outcomes than the others, varenicline monotherapy or combinations of NRT, that can be considered first-line or preferred medication strategies. Varenicline has demonstrated superiority in efficacy over nicotine medication or bupropion. Combination of a nicotine patch with a short-acting NRT, such as a gum or lozenge, is also an effective strategy that improves outcomes compared with nicotine medication or bupropion monotherapy (Lindson et al. 2019a). Although most of the studies of these medications have been conducted with people who smoke cigarettes, we include limited data, if available, for other types of tobacco products.

Table 7–1 presents a medication algorithm for considering various treatment options. Varenicline monotherapy or combination therapies of NRT should be considered first for most tobacco users. As with any medication, selection can be impacted by a range of other clinical factors, including patient preference, availability and insurance coverage, and the potential for side effects. Other considerations may include patients' experience during previous quit attempts, medical and psychiatric comorbidities, and the severity of their TUD. These issues, which are summarized in Table 7–1, might lead clinicians to consider an alternative or second-line approach. Keep in mind, however, that these approaches should be based on clinical judgment and lack conclusive data from placebo-controlled trials. For example, emerging evidence for medication selection based on factors such as sex, genetics, and specific symptom or illness patterns is still being developed and is inconclusive in most cases.

An essential aspect of using these medications successfully in clinical practice is to provide patient education. This serves numerous purposes. Clear instructions on practical details, such as taking varenicline with food to reduce nausea or avoiding using oral nicotine products with acidic beverages (e.g., coffee), not only enhance the medication's effectiveness but also reduce the risk of side effects that might cause people to discontinue use. All health care providers, and not just the prescribers, should be familiar with uses of these medications because discussing them and optimizing their use is integrated

Table 7–1. Medication algorithm: clinical considerations for medication selection

For most tobacco users

Use first-line treatments: combination NRT (patch + short acting) or varenicline →	Unless other considerations, e.g., insurance coverage, patient preference

Factors that might result in consideration of an alternative or second-line approach*

Comorbid depression	Could also consider
	• Bupropion (with or without NRT)
	• Nortriptyline
Comorbid alcohol use disorder	Varenicline may reduce alcohol intake and craving
Smokeless tobacco use	Nicotine lozenge or varenicline may have advantage
Schizophrenia and psychotic disorder	Could also consider
	• Bupropion and nicotine combination
Individuals with Medicare insurance (no coverage of over-the-counter NRT)	Combination NRT with nicotine inhaler (requires prior authorization)
	Bupropion
Failed with first-line medications in past	Could also consider
	• Retrial of same medications
	• Higher dosage
	• Bupropion (with or without NRT)
	• Nortriptyline
	• Combination of varenicline and bupropion
	• Nicotine nasal spray

Table 7–1. Medication algorithm: clinical considerations for medication selection (*continued*)

Unreliable, transient, homeless, elevated suicide risk	Over-the-counter NRT
Pregnant	Single NRT
	Bupropion
Unwilling to stop, willing to reduce	NRT (single or combination)
	Varenicline
Women	Possible better outcomes with varenicline than NRT
Multiple substance withdrawal or severe withdrawal including agitation or severe insomnia	Could also consider • Clonidine

NRT = nicotine replacement therapy.

*Note that these are suggested approaches that rely on good clinical practices. Some may lack conclusive data from high-quality placebo-controlled trials.

into the counseling approach that helps people cope with withdrawal and craving symptoms. When providing treatment as a clinical team, various members can participate in and support medication education efforts. Tools such as handouts about the medication make it easier by providing patients with supplementary information and reinforcing concepts. Examples of such handouts can be found on the website for the Tobacco Cessation Training and Technical Assistance Center (TCTTAC; https://nyctcttac.org/tag/medication-handout) program in New York City.

Education about tobacco withdrawal symptoms is an important part of ensuring patients are using their medications correctly. Remind them that nicotine is highly physically and psychologically addictive when smoked and that to be successful at quitting, they must overcome both. Tobacco withdrawal symptoms can be subtle or hard to distinguish from other conditions, including depression and anxiety. Patients can monitor for symptoms of irritable or depressed mood, trouble sleeping/insomnia, feelings of frustration, difficulty concentrating, restlessness, slower heart rate, or increased hunger, which can be strong determinants of relapse back to smoking during early abstinence. Learning about the nature and duration of tobacco withdrawal symptoms helps patients understand that these are temporary and that they will get better during the first few weeks of abstinence. Many people relapse during the first 3 days because of withdrawal symptoms, and getting them over this "hump" is very important. They need to know that tobacco withdrawal can be relieved in large part by tobacco treatment medications and that some of the psychosocial approaches may even further minimize symptoms of withdrawal.

An additional and often forgotten aspect of patient education is to validate the clear need for medication, which may not be obvious because of false beliefs and stigma about substance use disorders (SUDs). Pharmacological treatments for TUD have been shown to reduce withdrawal symptoms and to increase the chances of quitting successfully, yet patients (and even health care professionals) remain ambivalent. Old ideas that tobacco users must quit on their own or "pull themselves up by their bootstraps" are counterproductive and do not apply. Such beliefs undermine the biological aspects of addiction as a chronic disease and can leave people feeling discouraged and ashamed. Similarly, people may think that they only need medications to get through the first few days of tobacco withdrawal or that using the least possible amount makes them better or more successful, when the exact opposite is true. No one expects to recover from other chronic diseases with minimal or no treatment. For other illnesses, such as hypercholesterolemia and hypertension, medications are taken in an open-ended way and without shame, although lifestyle changes also help. Education about addiction as a biological disease that benefits from medication treatment is an important part of using these treatments effectively. For example, better outcomes (fewer relapses back to smoking) are associated with longer durations of treatment (~6 months), and patients should be encouraged to complete the entire course of treatment whenever possible. Some people may benefit from even longer durations of treatment, although evidence is limited to support this as a routine practice.

Tobacco Treatment Medications

Nicotine Replacement Therapies

FDA-approved nicotine medications include patches, gums, lozenges, and nasal sprays. Nicotine inhalers and oral sprays are additional products not available in the United States, although they are used in other parts of the world. Remind patients that it is always safer to use NRT in lieu of tobacco because these products contain only nicotine and not the toxins and carcinogens found in tobacco products. On the risk continuum, they are also safer than electronic cigarettes that also deliver nicotine because, as pharmaceutical products, they must adhere to standards for manufacturing and processing. About 25% of NRT users continue to be abstinent from smoking at 6 months using one of these products, and all forms of NRT are similar in efficacy. Nicotine poses little risk to a tobacco user who is physiologically tolerant to it, and decades of research on nicotine has proven it has little to no cardiotoxicity and does not cause cancer. Nicotine has no clinically significant medication interactions, and patches, gums, and lozenge formulations are available over-the-counter (OTC) in the United States. Because the out-of-pocket cost of OTC preparations can be a barrier for low-income populations, many state Medicaid programs now cover these medications when prescribed by a physician. Medicaid expansion has been effective in increasing access to treatments to low-income populations and has contributed to more quit attempts (Bailey et al. 2020). The 2010 Affordable Care Act in the United States mandated coverage for these medications through most commercial insurance plans.

Psychoeducation can help patients maximize the effectiveness of NRT because most people take NRT at too low a dosage or for too short a time. NRT generally produces blood nicotine levels lower than those achieved from smoking, and taking two NRT products simultaneously provides better withdrawal and craving relief (Carpenter et al. 2013). Each cigarette smoked delivers from 1 mg to 3 mg of nicotine to the body. This can be used as a crude estimate for dosing because someone who smokes a pack a day might have an average nicotine intake of about 40 mg nicotine (range 20–60 mg), which is almost double the amount delivered from a full-strength (21 mg/24 hours) nicotine patch. Nicotine is not effectively delivered to the body as an oral medication due to first-pass metabolism, making nicotine pills, nicotine water, and other non-FDA-approved formulations inadequate. Dosing nicotine all day long produces better outcomes than using it only as needed for cravings because this provides a steady level of nicotine in the blood that helps minimize withdrawal symptoms.

Nicotine can cause irritation on the skin as a side effect of patch use or in the mouth or throat as an effect of oral products, but these reactions are typically mild. Nicotine toxicity is rare in anyone who is tolerant to nicotine from regular tobacco use. Symptoms of nicotine toxicity, when they do occur, are usually self-limited and can include nausea, dizziness, and, in more severe cases, vomiting. NRT products do not differ in their effects on withdrawal, urges to smoke, user satisfaction, or rates of abstinence, and abuse liability from all are low. They do differ in their tendency for side effects, with the nasal spray producing far more adverse effects than the other forms. Cost is generally higher with prescription NRT (nasal spray); lower-cost generics are available for patches, gums, and lozenges.

Nicotine Transdermal Patch

The nicotine transdermal patch is available OTC, is easy to use, and is associated with good compliance given its once-daily dosing (Table 7–2). Patches provide slow, transdermal delivery of nicotine, with peak concentrations achieved 2–6 hours after application and steady-state levels reached within 2–4 days. Users should wear the patch for 24 hours, even while they sleep, to provide continuous nicotine delivery and to reduce early-morning withdrawal symptoms. However, the patch can be removed at night if sleep disturbances occur. Because insomnia is also a nicotine withdrawal symptom, this can be difficult to differentiate from a true patch side effect, although vivid or abnormal dreams are often a direct result of the nicotine. Removing the patch at nighttime effectively reduces the dose by at least 30%, and it is generally recommended that the patch be worn throughout the night to receive

Table 7–2. Nicotine patch (over-the-counter or prescription)

Starting dose	21 mg for ≥10 cigarettes per day; 14 mg for <10 per day
Route	Nicotine agonist; transdermal delivery
Side effects	Skin irritation, itching, sleep disturbance, vivid dreams
Tips for optimal use	Adheres best to clean, dry skin; rotate application site to lessen skin irritation
	Can be continued at 21-mg dose for an extended time
	Leave patch on while sleeping (as tolerated) to avoid early-morning cravings and risk for relapse
	Starting patch use before quit date may enhance outcomes
	Continue for 3–6 months and taper only when cravings are manageable

the full benefit. As mentioned in the "Nicotine Replacement Therapies" section, patches can be associated with local skin irritation; this is minimized by rotating the patch site every day. Users sometimes experience a sense of tingling or itching at the patch site that is typically mild and is not a reason to discontinue use. Patches generally adhere well as long as the skin is clean and dry prior to application.

The 21-mg dose is more effective than the 14-mg dose for smoking cessation and can be recommended for anyone who smokes 10 cigarettes per day or more (Lindson et al. 2019a). There is no strict timeline for tapering the dose (from 21 mg to 14 mg and then 7 mg), and patients should be mostly free from cravings before considering dose reductions. This might mean that the 21-mg dose is continued for 8–12 weeks before any reduction is made, and longer use may be necessary.

Oral Nicotine Products (Gum, Lozenge, Inhaler, and Oral Spray)

Four NRT products (gum, lozenge, inhaler, and oral spray) deliver nicotine to the bloodstream transmucosally, through the lining of the mouth. Although referred to as oral products, they are not swallowed; the goal is to avoid too much nicotine from entering the stomach, which causes side effects such as dyspepsia and hiccups. These products are most effective when kept in the mouth for a significant time to allow the nicotine to be slowly released and absorbed through the lining of the cheek and mouth. Although effective, these medications are generally thought of as low nicotine delivery products because the nicotine from a single use is typically less than that from one cigarette. The minimum effective number of doses for these products is eight per day, yet people often use fewer, which is associated with worse outcomes. In addition to being low-delivery, the oral forms of NRT should not be used with beverages such as coffee or soda, which are acidic. Nicotine is best absorbed in an alkaline environment, and making the mouth acidic makes oral NRTs less effective. An advantage of the immediate-acting forms of NRT is that they provide immediate craving relief and can be used as a rescue medication to supplement the longer-acting patch. Oral NRT options available in the United States are gums and lozenges. Nicotine inhalers and oral sprays are available in other parts of the world.

Nicotine gum (Table 7–3) delivers nicotine through the mucosa of the mouth and comes in a 2-mg and a 4-mg preparation. Patients should be instructed to slowly chew the gum and to pause and hold

Table 7–3. Nicotine gum (over-the-counter or prescription)

Starting dose	4 mg for ≥10 cigarettes per day; 2 mg for <10 per day
Route	Nicotine agonist; oral mucosa
Side effects	Mouth irritation, heartburn and hiccups (from swallowing nicotine), jaw soreness
Tips for optimal use	Use throughout the day every 1–2 hours and more for cravings
	Chew slowly and pause intermittently to hold gum in the cheek
	Avoid using with coffee and soda at the same time
	Continue for 3–6 months

it in their cheek (called the "bite and park" technique) for maximal nicotine absorption and to minimize swallowing. Users can taste the peppery nicotine and often can tell when the gum has been fully exhausted of nicotine after about 15 minutes. The recommended dosing is to chew one or two pieces per hour. It is estimated that only 0.5–1 mg of nicotine is absorbed on average from the 2-mg and 4-mg gums, respectively, and using the higher-strength (4 mg) formulation may be associated with greater quitting success, especially for people who are more highly dependent on nicotine (Lindson et al. 2019a). Although package dosing is based on number of cigarettes per day, an alternate approach would be to recommend the higher-strength dose for most people because deriving adequate nicotine replacement from the gum can be challenging. Its advantage is in its situational use to cope with cravings, although underdosing and improper use are common and can undermine success. Nicotine gum is not recommended for people with poor dentition, dentures, or temporomandibular joint problems. Nicotine gum is available OTC and comes in flavors such as mint that make it more palatable.

The nicotine lozenge (Table 7–4) is available OTC and works similarly to nicotine gum. Like gum, the lozenge is available in two strengths, 2 mg and 4 mg. It is not chewed but dissolves slowly in the mouth, making it better for people with jaw or dental problems. As a newer product, the instructions for use are based on the time to first cigarette (TTFC; first after overnight abstinence) rather than cigarettes smoked per day, which makes good clinical sense. The user determines

Table 7–4. Nicotine lozenge (over-the-counter or prescription)

Starting dose	4 mg for those who smoke within 30 minutes of waking, 2 mg for those who smoke their first cigarette of the day >30 minutes after waking
Route	Nicotine agonist; oral mucosa
Side effects	Mouth irritation, heartburn, and hiccups (from swallowing nicotine)
Tips for optimal use	Use throughout the day every 1–2 hours and more for cravings
	Dissolves in the mouth; do not chew
	Avoid using with coffee and soda at the same time
	Continue for 3–6 months

which dose is appropriate for them based on their TTFC. Those who use tobacco in the first 30 minutes of awakening should opt for higher-strength (4 mg) preparations. In fact, the 4-mg dose can be recommended for most people. The advantages of the nicotine lozenge are that it can be used situationally to cope with withdrawal symptoms and that it is more discreet than gum. The recommended dose is one lozenge every 1–2 hours for at least the first 6 weeks. Then users can try to taper off the lozenges, although a strict taper is not necessary and can be adjusted to each person's needs. Possible side effects include nausea, hiccups, and heartburn. Lozenges are the only NRT product that has demonstrated efficacy in people who use smokeless tobacco (Ebbert et al. 2015).

The nicotine oral spray (Table 7–5) was presented to the FDA in 2019 but is not yet approved in the United States. It has been available OTC in Canada and Europe for several years and is similar to other forms of oral NRT. This spray delivers a fine mist to the oral mucosa, and the smaller droplet size may allow for more rapid absorption than other oral forms of nicotine and thus faster relief of cravings. A dose is one or two sprays into the mouth (with 140 doses per container). Dosing can be up to four times an hour or a maximum of 64 doses per day, but in clinical trials most people used it 10–14 times per day. Each spray delivers 1 mg nicotine, and despite its slightly more rapid delivery, it is not associated with escalating use or abuse. The solution contains a tiny amount of ethanol, similar to mouthwash, and some people in recovery

Table 7–5. Nicotine oral spray (not available in United States)

Starting dose	One or two sprays into mouth every 1–2 hours
Route	Nicotine agonist; oral mucosa
Side effects	Mouth irritation, heartburn, and hiccups (from swallowing nicotine)
Tips for optimal use	Use throughout the day every 1–2 hours and more for cravings
	Avoid using with coffee and soda at the same time.
	Try to avoid swallowing too much nicotine.
	Continue for 3–6 months.

from alcohol addiction may want to avoid it for this reason (with administration of the full 64 doses per day, a person ingests <1 tsp of alcohol). Side effects can include hiccups, headache, nausea, mouth/throat irritation, dyspepsia, and dizziness associated with swallowing too much nicotine.

The nicotine inhaler (Table 7–6) is a plastic mouthpiece tube with a replaceable nicotine cartridge inside that is available only with a doctor's prescription. Manufacturing was ended in the United States in 2023, presumably as a marketing choice and not as a safety decision because it is still available in other parts of the world. When users

Table 7–6. Nicotine inhaler (not available in United States)

Starting dose	10-mg cartridge; puff one cartridge for 20 minutes every 1–2 hours
Route	Nicotine agonist; oral mucosa
Side effects	Mouth irritation, heartburn and hiccups (from swallowing nicotine), cough
Tips for optimal use	Use throughout the day every 1–2 hours and more for cravings.
	Avoid using with coffee and soda at the same time.
	Puff gently and slowly into mouth.
	Continue for 3–6 months.

gently puff on the inhaler, the cartridge provides a nicotine vapor into the mouth. The person can puff for 20–30 minutes to allow the nicotine to be absorbed through the oral mucosa. Recommended usage is 6–16 cartridges per day. Unlike other inhalers, which deliver most of the medication to the lungs, the nicotine inhaler delivers most of the nicotine vapor to the mouth, making it pharmacologically similar to the gum and lozenge. Behaviorally, nicotine inhalers are the closest NRT product to smoking a cigarette, which some people find helpful. The most common side effects, especially when first using the inhaler, include coughing, throat irritation, and upset stomach.

Nicotine Nasal Spray

Nicotine nasal spray (Table 7–7) delivers nicotine quickly to the bloodstream because it is absorbed fairly quickly through the mucosal lining of the nose. The spray rapidly relieves withdrawal symptoms and offers patients a sense of control over their nicotine cravings. It was developed as an alternative to oral nicotine that could provide a higher daily nicotine dose replacement and potentially help the people most severely addicted to smoking. The spray is only available by prescription and has an 80% discontinuation rate because it is associated with many side effects, especially during early use. The most common of these include nasal irritation, runny nose, watery eyes, sneezing, throat irritation, and coughing. Some users develop tolerance to these side effects with continued use. Nicotine nasal sprays have more liability for long-term use compared with other NRTs because of the more rapid

Table 7–7. Nicotine nasal spray (prescription)

Starting dose	10-mL bottle; one spray into each nostril every 1–2 hours
Route	Nicotine agonist; nasal mucosa
Side effects	Nasal irritation, sneezing, cough, watery eyes, runny nose
Tips for optimal use	Use throughout the day every 1–2 hours and more for cravings
	Side effects will dissipate with time and continued use
	Continue for 3–6 months

absorption of nicotine. Side effects should be explained to patients before they begin using the nasal spray, and they should be strongly encouraged to continue using the spray for the first 2 weeks until the side effects subside and they become used to using this product to satisfy nicotine cravings.

Non-Nicotine Treatments

Bupropion

Bupropion SR (Table 7–8) is a nonsedating antidepressant classified as a norepinephrine and dopamine reuptake inhibitor. It was later discovered to be a noncompetitive nicotinic receptor antagonist (Slemmer et al. 2000). This may explain its efficacy for tobacco cessation, which is not observed with most other antidepressants. For tobacco cessation, a daily dose of 150 mg or 300 mg can be effective, and its overall effectiveness is similar to NRT. Bupropion is usually started about 2 weeks before the quit date, and it is recommended that patients continue taking bupropion SR for at least 12 weeks (3 months) after they quit smoking. The most common side effects of bupropion SR are dry mouth, insomnia (trouble sleeping), and headache. It is contraindicated in anyone with a seizure disorder or an eating disorder due to its increased potential to cause a seizure. Although bupropion can be an excellent choice for someone with depression who smokes, its ability to help people quit smoking is independent of its effect on depression, so it is also helpful as a smoking cessation aid for people without diagnosed depression.

Table 7–8. Bupropion SR or XL (prescription)

Starting dose	150–300 mg
Route	Exact mechanism unknown, but inhibits norepinephrine and dopamine reuptake; oral
Side effects	Headache, insomnia, agitation, dry mouth
Tips for optimal use	Take for 1–2 weeks prior to quitting
	Continue for 3–6 months
	Also effective as an antidepressant

Common adverse effects include dry mouth, headache, and insomnia. Bupropion is contraindicated in people with history of seizures or bulimia, although the risk for seizure from the SR formulation is estimated to be low overall (0.1%) (Holm and Spencer 2000). Bupropion is a strong cytochrome P450 2D6 (CYP2D6) inhibitor, which means that interactions with other medications metabolized by CYP2D6 and CYP2B6 are possible, although perhaps not always clinically significant. One exception is that bupropion can reduce the effectiveness of tamoxifen in the treatment of breast cancer. Bupropion at a daily dose of 300 mg is associated with the lowest reported weight gain linked to stopping smoking. Although the FDA reviewed data on the SR formulation when the medication was approved for smoking cessation, the extended-release (XL) once-daily dosing is likely bioequivalent and is often preferred in clinical practice because it may enhance compliance and reduce side effects.

Varenicline

Varenicline (Table 7–9), known as Chantix in the United States, is a partial agonist at $\alpha_4\beta_2$ nicotinic acetylcholine receptors, which are found in the ventral tegmental area of the brain involved in the biology of addiction. Varenicline has a higher affinity than nicotine at this receptor, blocking the effects of nicotine when a person uses tobacco. In this way, it diminishes the reward experienced from tobacco use. As a partial agonist at the nicotine receptor, varenicline promotes the release of small amounts of dopamine at the nucleus accumbens, although varenicline is not addicting. Through its partial agonist properties, it helps prevent tobacco withdrawal by maintaining tone in the mesolimbic pathway.

Varenicline is titrated to a dosage of 1 mg twice a day in the first week, and doses can be taken with food to reduce the main side effect of nausea. A reduced dosage of 0.5 mg twice daily may also be effective if dosing is limited by side effects or reduced renal clearance (Fouz-Rosón et al. 2017). Because varenicline is renally excreted from the body into the urine, it has no clinically significant hepatic medication interactions. Other side effects include constipation, insomnia, and abnormal dreams. These do not seem to be dose dependent.

This medication requires a doctor's prescription and is usually started 1 week before the patient's planned quit date. Varenicline is the most effective medication treatment for smoking cessation when used as a monotherapy. This was shown in several studies, including

Table 7–9. Varenicline (prescription)

Starting dose	0.5–1.0 mg bid; titration in week 1 to dosage of 1 mg bid
Route	Nicotinic partial agonist; oral
Side effects	Headache, insomnia, agitation, dry mouth
Tips for optimal use	Take for 1–2 weeks prior to quitting
	Continue for 3–6 months
	No clinically significant medication interactions

the Evaluating Adverse Events in a Global Smoking Cessation Study (EAGLES), which is discussed in detail later (see "Clinical Focus" subsection) (Anthenelli et al. 2016). The EAGLES included people both with and without psychiatric illnesses who also smoked, making it highly generalizable. Many studies have validated varenicline's efficacy and safety, and it is not associated with more moderate to severe neuropsychiatric side effects than either bupropion or nicotine patch or placebo treatment (Thomas et al. 2015). A recent study demonstrated it was effective in African Americans who smoked, many of whom smoked fewer than 10 cigarettes per day (Cox et al. 2022). Varenicline has also demonstrated efficacy for quitting smokeless tobacco use (Schwartz et al. 2016). Studies show higher-than-usual dosages of varenicline may be effective in those who do not initially respond (Cinciripini et al. 2024).

Combination Treatments and Advanced Pharmacology

Studies indicate that combinations of two or more NRTs are more effective in reducing tobacco withdrawal symptoms and helping people successfully quit smoking (Lindson et al. 2019a). FDA guidelines were updated in April 2013 to support the safety of using combination NRT (see www.federalregister.gov/documents/2013/04/02/2013-07528 /modifications-to-labeling-of-nicotine-replacement-therapy-products -for-over-the-counter-human-use). A typical combination includes a long-lasting NRT such as a nicotine patch combined with an immediate-acting NRT to manage cravings. A full-strength (21 mg) patch may be insufficient in controlling nicotine withdrawal and urges in a sizable group of people. Supplementation of a long-acting patch with a short-acting NRT has advantages over using a single product. This combination delivers a higher dose and provides immediate craving relief in an as-needed manner. It also allows the user to titrate to the exact dose that works for them, which may vary on different days and in different situations. The more rapid (generally 10 minutes or less) nicotine supplementation from a short-acting NRT acts as a rescue medicine, with a behavioral component that helps people overcome feelings of withdrawal or cravings. Most combination NRT studies have evaluated nicotine gum or lozenge use with the patch; however, any combination would be expected to yield similar results. Whether using multiple NRTs (three products) offers an additional advantage is unclear, although some people prefer using different NRTs in different settings, such as a patch at work, a lozenge in the morning, and so on. This type of pattern does not cause toxicity and generally is not cause for concern. Studies of wearing two or more patches often fail to demonstrate enhanced efficacy in clinical trials, perhaps because the passive delivery of nicotine from the patch does not allow for optimal craving relief (Brokowski et al. 2014). This multiple-patch strategy is used much less often, although it can be potentially helpful for people who smoke very heavily (i.e., ≥40 cigarettes per day).

Combinations of bupropion and NRT are safe and well tolerated, although research studies have not always demonstrated this combination to be better than either nicotine patch or bupropion alone. However, using this combination is not unreasonable and can make clinical sense, especially if the patient has comorbid depression or has had another strong mood component during prior quit attempts. A triple combination (bupropion plus combination NRT) yielded better quit rates compared with patch alone in one randomized trial of people who smoked who were also medically ill (Steinberg et al. 2009).

Varenicline is not recommended for use in combination with NRT. Because varenicline blocks the nicotine receptor, no additional benefit is expected with supplemental nicotine, and this can worsen nausea and insomnia side effects. Several studies have evaluated this combination, and current evidence does not support this practice (Baker et al. 2021). Some have postulated a possible benefit in people who are severely dependent who may not experience complete nicotine receptor blockade with varenicline alone.

Combinations of varenicline and bupropion have been examined in a few clinical trials. Most, but not all, have shown a benefit compared with varenicline alone (Rose and Behm 2014). This combination is also safe and well tolerated because varenicline has no known medication interactions. A recent meta-analysis of four randomized controlled trials including more than 1,200 people who smoked showed that combination varenicline and bupropion significantly improved the abstinence rate at the end of treatment compared with varenicline alone. This benefit was seen mostly in people who smoked heavily and were highly dependent. The combination is associated with more side effects, including anxiety and insomnia, but is a reasonable approach to consider as a second- or third-line treatment or after an unsuccessful attempt with varenicline alone.

Treatment Duration and Relapse Prevention

The general recommendation is to use these medications for a duration of about 6 months following a quit attempt. Studies of this duration have shown it to be more effective in preventing relapse than shorter trials of 3 months or less. None of these medications is associated with long-term side effects, and someone may opt to use them longer than 6 months if they think it is necessary to keep them from resuming tobacco use. Studies of long-term NRT users report few, if any, health risks. Long-term use is not equivalent to having an SUD because although modest psychological or physiological dependence may occur, problematic use such as escalating, uncontrolled, or compulsive use is rarely evidenced.

One study in people with schizophrenia or bipolar disorder who smoked showed that taking varenicline for 12 months (vs. 3 months) reduced relapses back to smoking (Evins et al. 2014). An interesting aspect of this study was that many participants relapsed when the medication with withdrawn at 12 months, suggesting that even longer durations of treatment may be beneficial.

Other Issues

Metabolic Factors

Pharmacogenomics (sometimes called *pharmacogenetics*) is a field of research that studies how a person's genes affect how they respond to medications. Its goal is to help doctors select the medications and dosages best suited for each person. The rate of nicotine metabolism in the body predicts smoking behavior, ability to quit, and how well someone might respond to NRT in a quit attempt (Siegel et al. 2020; West et al. 2011). The nicotine metabolite ratio is a genetically informed biomarker that shows the activity of the nicotine metabolizing enzyme CYP2A6. It is a ratio of two nicotine metabolites (3'hydroxycotinine [3HC] and cotinine) taken from a saliva or plasma sample and does not require genotyping. Slow metabolizers have a protective effect in that they tend to smoke fewer cigarettes per day and are more likely to have never smoked or to have formerly smoked than fast metabolizers. One study showed that varenicline was more efficacious than nicotine patch in normal and fast metabolizers but not in slow metabolizers (Lerman et al. 2015). A high nicotine metabolite ratio was seen in a study of people with bipolar disorder who smoked; this likely was due to psychiatric medications that caused liver induction (Williams et al. 2012b). The impact of rapid nicotine metabolism on smoking behavior in people with bipolar disorder is not known. Although only used in research studies to date, nicotine metabolite ratios could become more widely available in the future and help in making clinical decisions about optimal pharmacotherapy treatments.

Weight Gain

One of the most common concerns around quitting smoking is weight gain. The large majority of people attempting to quit smoking who gain weight do so over the first few months after quitting, but many later lose much or all of this weight. Even though the health benefits of stopping smoking clearly outweigh the health risks of weight gain, fear of weight gain is a major deterrent to smoking cessation, especially among women. Use of tobacco treatment medications is associated with reduced or delayed weight gain and is another advantage of using this evidence-based approach. Intense efforts to control weight gain by dieting during abstinence may increase stress and cause relapse back to smoking because trying to stop using tobacco and make major dietary changes at the same time may be just too difficult. Patients should be encouraged to increase their physical activity, learn healthy eating strategies, and tolerate a moderate amount of weight gain that they can work on losing later rather than dieting now.

Medications for obesity and type II diabetes, known as glucagon-like peptide (GLP)-1 analogs, are being investigated as possible treatments for SUDs. They impact the mesolimbic dopamine system and have been found in animal studies to reduce intake of alcohol, nicotine, and other substances (Klausen et al. 2022). Preliminary studies in humans have been mixed, but these compounds, in addition to reducing craving and improving abstinence, have the potential to reduce the weight gain associated with quitting smoking (Yammine et al. 2021).

Treatments for People Who Are Not Immediately Ready to Quit Smoking

Pretreatment

All tobacco treatment medications can reduce the enjoyment of smoking as well as the nicotine withdrawal symptoms, making them helpful even in people who are not immediately ready to quit smoking. The benefits of using these medications prior to the quit date include becoming familiar with dosing and use and evaluating for tolerability and the potential for side effects. It also allows the medication to reach steady-state levels, which may take several days, ensuring the person receives a full dose at the timing of their quit attempt. Pretreatment with varenicline or bupropion is typically recommended for 10–14 days. Use of the patch has also been studied in combination with NRT, and some studies show a benefit from 7-day patch pretreatment while the person is still smoking (Lindson et al. 2019a). Most of these studies have only evaluated the patch. Although considered off-label use, this approach makes clinical sense because starting the patch on the quit date would mean the person would not receive the full nicotine dose until 6 hours after application, which may not be enough time to prevent relapse and may undermine the quit attempt due to nicotine withdrawal symptoms. Some studies pretreated participants with the nicotine patch for an even longer duration (2–4 weeks).

Using tobacco treatment medications while still smoking is a safe practice, even with NRT. The primary side effect from smoking while using NRT is mild toxicity (i.e., nausea), which is usually self-limited and might include feeling nauseated or dizzy. FDA guidelines were updated in April 2013 to support the safety of encouraging patients to continue use of NRT when smoking small amounts or for longer periods of time.

Smoking Reduction Strategies

Pharmacotherapy can also be effective for helping people who are not immediately ready to stop smoking. Overall, the evidence shows that "abrupt quitting" on a target quit date is more successful for people who are interested in quitting completely (Lindson et al. 2019b), and this is encouraged on the labeling for all of the medications. However, for those who are unwilling or not ready to quit abruptly, reduction is a reasonable option. People who successfully reduce their smoking amount often lower their level of dependence over time, and thus have higher rates of subsequently quitting. Generally, people are willing to try to cut down on their smoking even if they are not willing to quit completely, which allows for more individuals to become engaged in tobacco treatment. In this way, reduction strategies are consistent with other motivational approaches that allow the patient to determine the goals. A Cochrane Review of 51 trials involving more than 22,000 participants found evidence that reducing smoking with pharmacotherapy can be an effective strategy (Lindson et al. 2019b). Quantifying smoking reduction with biomarkers such as carbon monoxide or nicotine metabolite levels is more reliable than measures of cigarettes per day.

Smoking reduction strategies are generally more successful when done in conjunction with medications, which presumably reduce withdrawal symptoms to a tolerable level and minimize smoking compensation. Success in reducing the amount of smoking may lead to a greater sense of control and to subsequent greater motivation for eventually quitting and can be viewed as a harm reduction strategy. Tobacco treatment medications reduce the pleasure of smoking, which may also contribute to less smoking over time and to higher subsequent odds of quitting long-term. In routine medical care for other chronic health conditions, treatments are generally provided routinely, at the time of diagnosis, and are not based on an individual's motivation to change, even though many of these conditions also have a significant behavioral component (e.g., dietary guidelines for hypertension or non-insulin-dependent diabetes mellitus). In these cases, medical treatment is not withheld even if patients are not willing to comply with dietary restrictions. Medications for TUD have great potential to help a range of tobacco users and similarly should not be restricted to only those immediately wanting to quit or participate in counseling.

Several trials have tested NRT as an intervention to assist with smoking reduction. Use of NRT is associated with significant reductions in smoking, as well as with an increased likelihood of quitting smoking in populations currently unable or unwilling to quit, although this is considered an off-label use (Lindson-Hawley et al. 2016). An analysis of people using NRT for 6–18 months while smoking revealed quit rates of 7% and very low rates of adverse events (mainly nausea) (Moore et al. 2009).

Varenicline is also effective for smoking reduction. A large trial of varenicline versus placebo for 24 weeks in people not willing or able to immediately quit smoking demonstrated that use of varenicline was associated with much higher rates of abstinence from smoking at 6 months and 12 months (Ebbert et al. 2015). Varenicline reduction strategies have been so successful that they are part of the on-label FDA-approved usage recommendations. Clinicians should prescribe varenicline and encourage patients to reduce their smoking by 50% within the first 4 weeks and then by 50% more in the following 4 weeks, with the goal of reaching complete abstinence by 12 weeks.

Periods of Temporary Abstinence

Nicotine withdrawal emerges within hours of someone's last use of tobacco and can cause discomfort, including urges to smoke, restlessness, or feeling angry or irritable in addition to cognitive effects such as poor attention. Nicotine medication can be used safely and should be encouraged during these periods of temporary abstinence (Foulds 2010). Not only will this lessen the withdrawal symptoms but it also may provide the person with a positive experience using NRT that can facilitate future attempts at tobacco reduction or cessation.

Psychiatric patients who have higher levels of tobacco use experience significant tobacco withdrawal symptoms during periods of abstinence that may complicate their mental health care. Withdrawal symptoms are somewhat nonspecific and overlap with symptoms of depression, anxiety disorders, and other SUDs. Failing to recognize tobacco withdrawal symptoms may lead to overuse of other psychiatric medications to reduce agitation, anxiety, or restlessness. People who smoked and did not receive NRT during an inpatient psychiatric stay were more likely to sign out against medical advice, underscoring the clinical importance of addressing tobacco withdrawal (Prochaska et al. 2004). Agitation was reduced to a clinically significant degree in a study of people with schizophrenia who smoked who received a 21-mg nicotine patch in an emergency department setting (Allen et al. 2011). This low-cost strategy reduces suffering and optimizes other mental health care and should be done routinely in settings that detain patients or restrict their tobacco use for periods of 4 hours or more, including screening centers or day-treatment programs.

Other Treatments

None of the treatments described in the following sections is currently FDA approved, although they have some evidence of efficacy.

Nortriptyline

Nortriptyline is an older tricyclic antidepressant found to be as effective for quitting smoking as NRT (Howes et al. 2020). It is generally not used and is considered a second- or third-line treatment because it has significant side effects, including weight gain, sedation, and orthostatic hypotension. It can be used if the person prefers it or has a history of depression. Nortriptyline is dosed in the same way as an antidepressant, and serum drug levels can be helpful in determining an adequate dosage. Given the availability of more effective medications with less common or severe side effects, nortriptyline is not often used as an aid to smoking cessation.

Cytisine

Although not available in the United States at this time, cytisine is an OTC formulation that has been used in Eastern Europe for decades (sold as Tabex). Cytisine (also known as cytisinicline) is a plant derivative that works as a nicotinic partial agonist and has a molecular structure similar to that of nicotine and acetylcholine. The development of varenicline was based on the cytisine structure. Several recent trials support its efficacy as an effective smoking cessation medication. In an open-label study, it was associated with higher quit rates than the nicotine patch (Walker et al. 2014). Another showed cytisine to have outcomes comparable with those of varenicline (6 months of continuous abstinence: 11.7% cytisine vs. 13.3% varenicline) (Courtney et al. 2021). The recommended dosage for cytisine is 1.5 capsules taken six times daily initially and then gradually reduced over the 25-day course. Tolerability of cytisine is comparable with that of other treatments, and the most common side effects are nausea, insomnia, and abnormal dreams (Courtney et al. 2021). In countries where cytisine is approved, it may have the advantage of being less expensive than other treatments. A recent study evaluated 6-week and 12-week cytisine use (vs. placebo) in a revised dosing paradigm (3-mg tablet dosed three times daily). Both 6-week and 12-week treatments resulted in greater success in quitting smoking than placebo (Rigotti et al. 2023).

Participants receiving cytisine had six- to eightfold higher odds of continuous smoking abstinence at the end of treatment than participants receiving placebo plus behavioral support. Some people quit after the first 6 weeks of treatment, suggesting that longer durations may be helpful and that treatment should continue even in those who are not able to quit in the first week. Cytisine is being evaluated for potential market approval in the United States and, if approved as an OTC treatment, has the potential to reach many tobacco users.

Clonidine

Clonidine is listed as a second-line treatment in the U.S. Public Health Service Guidelines, but it is rarely used since the emergence of more effective agents. It is an α-adrenergic agonist used in the treatment of hypertension that is sometimes also used for opioid withdrawal management because it reduces heart rate and response to catecholamines. Side effects include hypotension and sedation.

Failed Clinical Trials

Other medications have been studied and determined to be ineffective for smoking cessation. These include naltrexone (opioid antagonist), selegiline (monoamine oxidase inhibitor), anxiolytics, lobeline, N-acetylcysteine, St. John's wort, and selective serotonin reuptake inhibitors (Cahill et al. 2013; Howes et al. 2020). Current evidence for mecamylamine in combination with NRT is inconclusive.

Clinically Significant Interactions

Tobacco smoke is a potent inducer of the CYP1A2 isoenzyme, reducing the serum level and presumed effectiveness of important medications. This includes commonly used antipsychotics and antidepressants such as clozapine, olanzapine, and fluvoxamine and other medications such as theophylline (Oliveira et al. 2017). Smoking results in the need for higher medication dosages and the potential for medication toxicity during a quit attempt. The major effect is not due to nicotine but to the inhaled polycyclic aromatic hydrocarbons in smoke. Nicotine is metabolized by a different enzyme (CYP2A6) and has no effect on other medication levels. A comprehensive list of these interactions is shown in Chapter 5, Table 5–1.

Clinical Focus: Neuropsychiatric Safety and Efficacy of Varenicline, Bupropion, and Nicotine Patch in People With and Without Psychiatric Disorders Who Smoke

Varenicline was approved by the FDA (Chantix) and the European Commission (Champix) in 2006 for use as an aid to smoking cessation therapy. By 2008, case reports had been made of individuals who had neuropsychiatric symptoms including changes in behavior, agitation, depressed mood, or suicidal thoughts or behavior when taking the medication. Although causality was not established and this effect had not been seen in earlier clinical trials of more than 5,000 people that compared it with placebo, both varenicline and bupropion were given a black box warning in 2009 to warn of possible serious neuropsychiatric effects.

The EAGLES (Anthenelli et al. 2016) was designed to address substantial concerns raised about the neuropsychiatric safety of varenicline and bupropion. The FDA required the makers of these medications to conduct a sufficiently large randomized trial to provide greater clarity on their potential safety risks. The EAGLES is a seminal work as a very large double-blind, triple-dummy, active- and placebo-controlled randomized trial in people with and without a psychiatric disorder who smoked. The study recruited individuals with and without mental illness who wanted to try to quit smoking from 140 study centers in 16 countries. Participants with mental illness (n=4,074) were stable outpatients with mood disorders (71%; depression or bipolar disorder), anxiety disorders (19%; mainly generalized anxiety disorder, panic disorder, or PTSD), or psychotic disorders (9%; schizophrenia). Diagnoses were confirmed with the Structured Clinical Interview for DSM-5 (SCID). Participants without mental illness (n=3,984) also had the absence of diagnosis confirmed with the SCID. Participants were excluded if they had had an alcohol use disorder or SUD in the past 12 months.

Participants were randomly assigned to receive either varenicline 1 mg twice a day, bupropion SR 150 mg twice a day, transdermal nicotine patch 21 mg/day with taper, or placebo for a 12-week treatment phase followed by a 12-week follow-up (no medication) phase. In this triple-dummy design, everyone took two pills and wore a patch daily; these consisted of either one active treatment (varenicline, bupropion, or nicotine) and two placebos (for the others), or three placebos. Participants were asked to complete up to 15 face-to-face visits and 11 telephone visits during the 24-week trial. Participants used an average of 21 cigarettes per day, with an average Fagerström Test for Cigarette Dependence score of 5.8, and 82% had made at least one previous attempt to quit. Among those who smoked and had mental illness, 49% were taking psychiatric medications at baseline, 34% had a history of suicidal ideation, and 13% had a history of past suicidal behavior.

The primary outcome of the EAGLES was a composite measure of neuropsychiatric side effects that was assessed weekly. This comprehensive measure could include any of the following experiences: anxiety, depression, feeling abnormal, hostility, agitation, aggression, delusions, hallucinations, homicidal ideation, mania, panic, paranoia, psychosis, suicidal behavior, suicidal ideation, and completed suicide. The primary efficacy endpoint for smoking cessation was the self-report of continuous abstinence rate for weeks 9–12, confirmed by an exhaled carbon monoxide reading of 10 ppm or less. The overall incidence of the neuropsychiatric events endpoint was similar across the four treatment groups: varenicline 4.0% (80 of 2,016 participants), bupropion 4.5% (90 of 2,006 participants), nicotine patch 3.9% (78 of 2,022 participants), and placebo 3.7% (74 of 2,014 participants). More neuropsychiatric adverse events were reported in the psychiatric cohort (5.8%) than in the nonpsychiatric cohort (2.1%), but there were no significant medication effects. Side effects reported by the active treatment groups more than the placebo group were nausea (varenicline 25%), insomnia (bupropion 12%), and abnormal dreams (nicotine patch 12%).

Varenicline showed superior efficacy to bupropion and nicotine patch. All three medication treatments were significantly better than the group receiving only placebos (counseling alone). In both the mental illness and non–mental illness cohorts, varenicline was superior to either bupropion or patch, which had similar efficacy to each other (Figure 7–1). Participants with mental illness achieved lower abstinence rates overall than those in the nonpsychiatric cohort. The study did not show a significant increase in neuropsychiatric adverse events attributable to varenicline or bupropion relative to nicotine patch or placebo. Varenicline was more effective than placebo, nicotine patch, and bupropion in helping people achieve abstinence from smoking. This was true for both groups, with and without mental illness.

This study is important for many reasons. The triple-dummy design allowed for conclusive evidence regarding the lack of moderate to serious neuropsychiatric side effects from varenicline. Experiencing symptoms of anxiety, depression, or agitation during a quit attempt might be attributed to nicotine withdrawal, underlying illness, or other reason. Rates of these experiences were not different in groups receiving the other medications (bupropion or nicotine patch) or only placebos. Having anxiety at baseline (regardless of having a diagnosis of anxiety disorder) predicted reporting a serious neuropsychiatric side effect. The higher overall occurrence of these symptoms among participants with mental illness who smoked is also not surprising and reflects the nature of the underlying psychiatric disorders. Predictors of moderate to severe neuropsychiatric side effects in the study included having current anxiety or prior suicidal ideation at baseline and being White (but did not vary by medication group). Among those with mental illness, additional predictors included female sex, younger age, history of SUD, and greater severity of nicotine dependence or mental illness (but not medication type). This evidence, as well as other meta-analyses, led the FDA and the European Commission to remove the black box warning from the labeling instructions in 2016. This study also provided valuable information about smoking cessation in individuals with known mental illness, a population that had previously been excluded from studies, and yielded a large dataset for secondary analyses. Under the same controlled conditions, these individuals are less successful in their quit attempt compared with those without mental illness, although other baseline characteristics are similar.

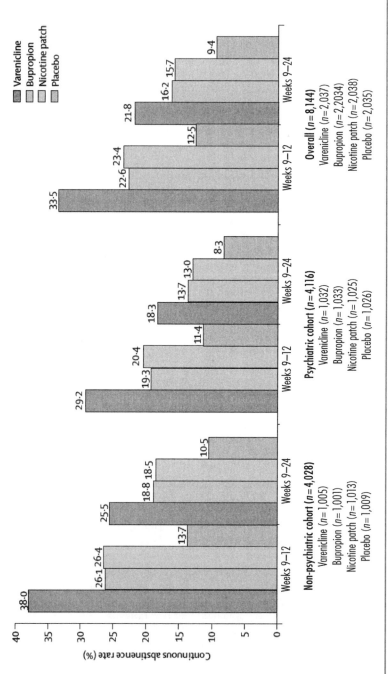

Figure 7–1. Continuous abstinence rates in the Evaluating Adverse Events in a Global Smoking Cessation Study (EAGLES).

Source. Anthenelli et al. 2016.

Induction of the cytochrome P450 system by tobacco is consistent with clinical epidemiological findings that people who smoke are more likely to be taking higher medication dosages. Increased dosages of medications often lead to more side effects and to higher costs because many medications are priced higher with increasing dosage. During periods of abstinence, enzyme activity of CYP1A2 can return to normal levels, perhaps in a few days, although this is not well studied. This decline can result in potential toxicity of any affected medications that have been dosed higher due to the person smoking. Despite these presumed fluctuations, many medications seem to be well tolerated, and changes may not be noticed, although sedation or other side effects may occur. A few case reports have been made of clozapine toxicity and seizure during early tobacco abstinence, and patients taking clozapine should be monitored closely for possible toxicity (Zullino et al. 2002). Measuring serum clozapine levels may be helpful, and dosage reduction could be needed.

Cigarette smoke also increases the metabolism of caffeine, which lowers serum caffeine levels (Zevin and Benowitz 1999). Thus, to maintain the same stimulating effects of caffeine (e.g., alertness), people who smoke likely compensate by increasing their caffeine intake (i.e., consuming more caffeinated beverages). Again, during early abstinence, enzyme activity of CYP1A2 can return to normal levels and result in potential toxicity with high caffeine intake, although this also has not been well studied. Complaints of insomnia and irritability during the first few days of smoking abstinence could theoretically be due, at least in part, to caffeine toxicity, and it makes clinical sense to recommend lowering caffeine intake during a quit attempt.

In contrast to tobacco smoke, nicotine is metabolized by different hepatic enzymes: CYP2A6 and CYP2B6. Nicotine has no clinically significant medication interactions, although oral contraceptives and hepatic inducers, including carbamazepine, have been known to increase its metabolism and result in lower serum nicotine levels (Williams et al. 2010). Varenicline is excreted mostly unchanged in the urine and not by the liver; thus, it has no clinically significant medication interactions. Bupropion is a strong CYP2D6 inhibitor, which means that interactions with other medications metabolized by CYP2D6 and CYP2B6 are possible, although perhaps not always clinically significant. One exception is that bupropion can reduce the effectiveness of tamoxifen in the treatment of breast cancer. These potential medication interactions are summarized in Table 7–10.

Table 7–10. Clinically significant interactions

Product	Route of metabolism	Clinically significant interactions
Nicotine and nicotine replacement therapy	Liver, CYP2A6	None
Bupropion	Liver, CYP2B6, CYP2D6 inhibitor	Potential, but modest clinical significance
Varenicline	Kidney, excreted in urine	None
Tobacco smoke tar	Liver, CYP1A2 inducer	Many; reduces level of olanzapine, clozapine, tricyclic antidepressants, caffeine, duloxetine, mirtazapine, and fluvoxamine

Medication Considerations for Special Populations

Behavioral Health Comorbidity

Studies of tobacco users with mental health comorbidity show that, in general, these treatments work and are well tolerated. Some evidence indicates that the overall success rate in a given attempt may be lower in this population compared with people without mental illness. Many studies have shown no worsening of depression or psychosis symptoms when people try to quit smoking. Studies have also been conducted in people with various SUDs, and these also show that medications are effective and well tolerated. Individuals who are in recovery from substances for 1 year or longer generally can be as successful as others in quitting; less is known about people in early recovery who try to quit. Tobacco treatment considerations for diagnostic subgroups of mental illnesses or SUDs, including issues such as timing of treatment, are discussed in more detail in Chapter 11.

Neuropsychiatric Side Effects and Varenicline

Varenicline has been studied extensively in terms of its impact on mental health symptoms and in populations with known psychiatric disorders. No evidence from randomized, double-blind, placebo-controlled trials has shown varenicline to cause suicide, suicidal ideation, depression, irritability, or aggression (Cahill et al. 2016). Smaller studies using a variety of symptom measure scales in populations with major depression, schizophrenia, and bipolar disorder also showed no evidence of suicide and no worsening of the primary illness (Anthenelli et al. 2013; Chengappa et al. 2014; Williams et al. 2012a). Much of this evidence comes from the large, multisite EAGLES, which studied more than 8,000 people who smoked, including more than 4,000 who also had SCID-confirmed psychiatric disorders (mood, anxiety, and psychotic disorders; also discussed in Table 5–1 and the "Clinical Focus" section earlier in this chapter). In addition to confirming the superiority of varenicline over placebo, nicotine patch, and bupropion, the EAGLES confirmed the absence of severe neuropsychiatric side effects, with no differences between medication groups (Anthenelli et al. 2016).

In 2009, the FDA issued the black box warning in response to clinical reports of suicidal thoughts, hostility, and agitation. This came from case report data and not from randomized trials with placebo groups. The warning was removed in 2016 after several studies, including the EAGLES, failed to show an association between varenicline use and moderate to severe neuropsychiatric side effects. Neuropsychiatric side effects were defined broadly in the EAGLES to include symptoms of anxiety/panic, depression, hostility, agitation, aggression, delusions, psychosis, hallucinations, paranoia, homicidal or suicidal ideation, and mania. Given this wealth of safety information, policies restricting varenicline use, especially among those with behavioral health conditions, should be eliminated because the risk of tobacco far outweighs the potential risk from medications.

The incidence of moderate to severe neuropsychiatric side effects was higher among people who smoked who were in the psychiatric cohort (5.9%) than those in the nonpsychiatric cohort (2.1%), although medication group was not a factor (Anthenelli et al. 2019). In the total sample, individuals with current symptoms of anxiety or prior suicidal ideation/behavior were more likely to experience moderate to severe neuropsychiatric side effects. Among the patients with psychiatric comorbidity, having more severe nicotine dependence or psychiatric illness was also predictive of a neuropsychiatric side effect, suggesting that in some cases these symptoms may represent tobacco withdrawal or other symptoms of mental illness.

Large database studies have also been conducted to examine effects on population health. Use of varenicline is associated with reduced risk for hospitalization for a cardiovascular problem or psychiatric illness (Carney et al. 2021). Varenicline has been studied in SUD populations and found to be safe and effective (Guo et al. 2021). In addition, varenicline may impact alcohol intake and drinking outcomes by modulating reward in the reward pathway (Oon-Arom et al. 2019; Vatsalya et al. 2015). Studies of NRT and bupropion in populations with mental illness or an SUD have been published, in addition to the EAGLES study, that demonstrate that these treatments are safe and well tolerated.

Pregnancy

Rates of smoking are about 7% among pregnant females in the United States, but rates are higher among those with lower socioeconomic status or comorbid mental illness or SUD (Alshaarawy et al. 2021; Goodwin et al. 2017). Females with depression and low social support have more difficulty quitting smoking during pregnancy. One study showed that one-third of pregnant females who smoked were also using other drugs, mostly cannabis (Gaalema et al. 2013). Having depression and anxiety also predicts smoking relapse postpartum (Correa-Fernandez et al. 2012; Park et al. 2009). Smoking reduces a person's chances of getting pregnant, in addition to increasing their risk for pregnancy complications (U.S. Department of Health and Human Services 2020). Tobacco smoke also harms offspring before and after they are born, making the need for cessation highly important.

There is conflicting evidence from clinical trials as to whether NRT or bupropion increases abstinence rates in pregnancy, although clinically their use makes sense for those who are unable to quit smoking on their own. Factors possibly contributing to lower efficacy during pregnancy include poor adherence to medications, increased metabolic rate, and lower doses of NRT used. Studies of NRT and bupropion show no evidence of adverse effects on children's health, and some show evidence of better outcomes, including higher birth weight (Patnode et al. 2021). Use of these medications can be considered during pregnancy because the greatest risk to the unborn fetus is from the lack of oxygen and the toxin exposure from cigarette smoke. In a clinical setting, it is reasonable to discuss the risks and benefits and to initiate a trial of pharmacotherapy during pregnancy in anyone who has been unable to quit smoking on their own or with counseling alone. The American College of Obstetricians and Gynecologists recommends that use of NRT be undertaken with close supervision and after careful consideration and discussion with the patient about the known risks of continued smoking and the possible risks of treatment (American College of Obstetricians and Gynecologists Committee on Obstetric Practice 2020).

Accidental exposure to NRT, bupropion, or varenicline during pregnancy does not seem to be associated with birth defects or other negative consequences, although varenicline should be avoided because the data are limited and safety has not been established.

Youth

There are limited studies of pharmacotherapy for smoking cessation in young people (age <20 years). No clear evidence has been found for the effectiveness of NRT, bupropion, or varenicline in this population (Fanshawe et al. 2017; Gray et al. 2019). In a trial of varenicline versus placebo, 59% of participants had a positive urine drug screen for cannabis at baseline, and this significantly reduced their likelihood of achieving abstinence from smoking (McClure et al. 2020). The complex issues surrounding tobacco, nicotine, and cannabis co-use are discussed in Chapter 11.

Other Biological Treatments for Tobacco Use Disorder

There has been growing interest in other biological treatments that hold promise for addictions, including TUD. These include transcranial magnetic stimulation (TMS), vaccines, and psychedelics. Vaccines that target nicotine and stimulate the immune system to produce specific antibodies are being investigated. Conceptually, vaccines for SUD would work by reducing delivery of the substance to the brain. Nicotine vaccines have been well tolerated in clinical trials, and antibody levels tend to decline slowly over months following administration (U.S. Department of Health and Human Services 2020). The efficacy of nicotine vaccines has not yet been established as an aid to smoking cessation or to relapse prevention, likely because they do not produce antibody levels high enough to be fully effective.

TMS is a noninvasive form of brain stimulation that uses magnetic pulses to stimulate nerve cells in the brain. These high-current pulses are delivered through a scalp-placed electromagnetic coil and passed into brain tissue in a targeted area. When performed repeatedly, TMS is a treatment for depression and is generally well tolerated, with few side effects. TMS also holds promise for the treatment of addictions by focusing on implicated areas such as the dorsolateral prefrontal cortex or insula. One randomized, sham-controlled study of 15 TMS sessions (five per week) found a higher 4-week rate of continuous abstinence from cigarettes and reduced craving compared with placebo (Zangen et al. 2021). This one study resulted in FDA approval of TMS for smoking cessation treatment, although access is still limited, and cost and acceptability may be real-world barriers. The impact of TMS on craving and relapse prevention is an area of interest for future study.

Interest has grown in the study of psychedelics as potential treatments for behavioral health conditions, including other SUDs. Two strategies often tested are the psychedelic model, which is intended to produce a single overwhelming experience, and the psycholytic model, in which lower doses are administered that may not be psychoactive. Psilocybin, which impacts serotonin-2A receptors, is being tested for treatment of alcohol use disorder and TUD. Epidemiological studies suggest an association between lifetime psilocybin use and lower rates of smoking (Jones et al. 2022). One open-label pilot study showed that two doses of psilocybin helped 15 of 16 people achieve abstinence (Johnson et al. 2014), but larger, placebo-controlled trials are needed. This study used moderate to high doses of psilocybin, and the quality of the mystical experience was linked to greater success in quitting smoking, suggesting that the spiritual and personal meanings of the experience matter (Garcia-Romeu et al. 2014).

Key Points

- Medications to treat nicotine addiction are a first-line treatment with a large evidence base demonstrating their safety and efficacy.

- Most people do not use these medications correctly, in a high enough dose or for a long enough time, which undermines success in a quit attempt. Providing education is essential to success.
- Nicotine replacement therapy, bupropion, and varenicline are all FDA approved and, in combination with counseling, yield the greatest success in quitting smoking.
- Nicotine medications are safe and well tolerated and should be dosed aggressively to reduce the nicotine withdrawal and craving symptoms that undermine quit attempts.
- Bupropion is a safe and well-tolerated treatment option. Its effect is independent of its effect on depression, and it may cause the least amount of weight gain during a quit attempt.
- Varenicline has demonstrated evidence of better efficacy than nicotine replacement or bupropion when used as a monotherapy. Considerable evidence, including the large EAGLES clinical trial, supports its safety and lack of serious neuropsychiatric side effects.
- Combination nicotine replacement therapy or varenicline should be considered first-line treatments with better outcomes than other medication options.
- Evidence for the use of cytisine as an aide to quitting smoking is growing, and it may be another option to consider in the future.
- Tobacco smoke causes reductions in the blood level of several commonly used medications and caffeine.
- In people who are not yet ready to quit smoking, tobacco treatment medications can help them reduce the amount they smoke per day and work toward eventual quitting by reducing withdrawal effects and blocking the enjoyment they typically receive from smoking.
- In populations where the evidence is limited, clinical judgment should err on the side of providing treatment whenever possible because the continued risks of smoking are nearly always worse than the potential risk from the specific treatment.

References

Allen MH, Debanné M, Lazignac C, et al: Effect of nicotine replacement therapy on agitation in smokers with schizophrenia: a double-blind, randomized, placebo-controlled study. Am J Psychiatry 168(4):395–399, 2011 21245085

Alshaarawy O, Roskos SE, Meghea CI: Tobacco cigarette and cannabis use among new mothers. Addiction 116(9):2572–2576, 2021 33314407

American College of Obstetricians and Gynecologists Committee on Obstetric Practice: Tobacco and nicotine cessation during pregnancy. ACOG Committee Opinion No 807. Obstet Gynecol 135(5):e221–e229, 2020

Anthenelli RM, Morris C, Ramey TS, et al: Effects of varenicline on smoking cessation in adults with stably treated current or past major depression: a randomized trial. Ann Intern Med 159(6):390–400, 2013 24042367

Anthenelli RM, Benowitz NL, West R, et al: Neuropsychiatric safety and efficacy of varenicline, bupropion, and nicotine patch in smokers with and without psychiatric disorders (EAGLES): a double-blind, randomised, placebo-controlled clinical trial. Lancet 387(10037):2507–2520, 2016 27116918

Anthenelli RM, Gaffney M, Benowitz NL, et al: Predictors of neuropsychiatric adverse events with smoking cessation medications in the randomized controlled EAGLES trial. J Gen Intern Med 34(6):862–870, 2019 30847828

Bailey SR, Marino M, Ezekiel-Herrera D, et al: Tobacco cessation in Affordable Care Act Medicaid expansion states versus non-expansion states. Nicotine Tob Res 22(6):1016–1022, 2020 31123754

Baker TB, Piper ME, Smith SS, et al: Effects of combined varenicline with nicotine patch and of extended treatment duration on smoking cessation: a randomized clinical trial. JAMA 326(15):1485–1493, 2021 34665204

Benowitz NL, Pipe A, West R, et al: Cardiovascular safety of varenicline, bupropion, and nicotine patch in smokers: a randomized clinical trial. JAMA Intern Med 178(5):622–631, 2018 29630702

Brokowski L, Chen J, Tanner S: High-dose transdermal nicotine replacement for tobacco cessation. Am J Health Syst Pharm 71(8):634–638, 2014 24688036

Cahill K, Stevens S, Perera R, et al: Pharmacological interventions for smoking cessation: an overview and network meta-analysis. Cochrane Database Syst Rev 2013(5):CD009329, 2013 23728690

Cahill K, Lindson-Hawley N, Thomas KH, et al: Nicotine receptor partial agonists for smoking cessation. Cochrane Database Syst Rev 2016(5):CD006103, 2016 27158893

Carney G, Maclure M, Malfair S, et al: Comparative safety of smoking cessation pharmacotherapies during a government-sponsored reimbursement program. Nicotine Tob Res 23(2):302–309, 2021 32484873

Carpenter MJ, Jardin BF, Burris JL, et al: Clinical strategies to enhance the efficacy of nicotine replacement therapy for smoking cessation: a review of the literature. Drugs 73(5):407–426, 2013 23572407

Chengappa KNR, Perkins KA, Brar JS, et al: Varenicline for smoking cessation in bipolar disorder: a randomized, double-blind, placebo-controlled study. J Clin Psychiatry 75(7):765–772, 2014 25006684

Cinciripini PM, Green CE, Shete S, et al: Smoking cessation after initial treatment failure with varenicline or nicotine replacement: a randomized clinical trial. JAMA 331(20):1722–1731, 2024 38696203

Correa-Fernández V, Ji L, Castro Y, et al: Mediators of the association of major depressive syndrome and anxiety syndrome with postpartum smoking relapse. J Consult Clin Psychol 80(4):636–648, 2012

Courtney RJ, McRobbie H, Tutka P, et al: Effect of cytisine vs varenicline on smoking cessation: a randomized clinical trial. JAMA 326(1):56–64, 2021 34228066

Cox LS, Nollen NL, Mayo MS, et al: Effect of varenicline added to counseling on smoking cessation among African American daily smokers: the Kick It at Swope IV randomized clinical trial. JAMA 327(22):2201–2209, 2022 35699705

Ebbert JO, Elrashidi MY, Stead LF: Interventions for smokeless tobacco use cessation. Cochrane Database Syst Rev 2015(10):CD004306, 2015 26501380

Evins AE, Cather C, Pratt SA, et al: Maintenance treatment with varenicline for smoking cessation in patients with schizophrenia and bipolar disorder: a randomized clinical trial. JAMA 311(2):145–154, 2014 24399553

Fanshawe TR, Halliwell W, Lindson N, et al: Tobacco cessation interventions for young people. Cochrane Database Syst Rev 11(11):CD003289, 2017 29148565

Foulds J: Use of nicotine replacement therapy to treat nicotine withdrawal syndrome and aid temporary abstinence. Int J Clin Pract 64(3):292–294, 2010 20456168

Fouz-Rosón N, Montemayor-Rubio T, Almadana-Pacheco V, et al: Effect of 0.5 mg versus 1 mg varenicline for smoking cessation: a randomized controlled trial. Addiction 112(9):1610–1619, 2017 28449281

Gaalema DE, Higgins ST, Pepin CS, et al: Illicit drug use among pregnant women enrolled in treatment for cigarette smoking cessation. Nicotine Tob Res 15(5):987–991, 2013

Garcia-Romeu A, Griffiths RR, Johnson MW: Psilocybin-occasioned mystical experiences in the treatment of tobacco addiction. Curr Drug Abuse Rev 7(3):157–164, 2014 25563443

Goodwin RD, Cheslack-Postava K, Nelson DB, et al: Smoking during pregnancy in the United States, 2005–2014: the role of depression. Drug Alcohol Depend 179:159–166, 2017 28783546

Gray KM, Baker NL, McClure EA, et al: Efficacy and safety of varenicline for adolescent smoking cessation: a randomized clinical trial. JAMA Pediatr 173(12):1146–1153, 2019 31609433

Guo K, Li J, Li J, et al: The effects of pharmacological interventions on smoking cessation in people with alcohol dependence: a systematic review and meta-analysis of nine randomized controlled trials. Int J Clin Pract 75(11):e14594, 2021 34228852

Holm KJ, Spencer CM: Bupropion: a review of its use in the management of smoking cessation. Drugs 59(4):1007–1024, 2000 10804045

Howes S, Hartmann-Boyce J, Livingstone-Banks J, et al: Antidepressants for smoking cessation. Cochrane Database Syst Rev 4(4):CD000031, 2020 32319681

Johnson MW, Garcia-Romeu A, Cosimano MP, et al: Pilot study of the 5-HT2AR agonist psilocybin in the treatment of tobacco addiction. J Psychopharmacol 28(11):983–992, 2014 25213996

Jones G, Lipson J, Nock MK: Associations between classic psychedelics and nicotine dependence in a nationally representative sample. Sci Rep 12(1):10578, 2022 35732796

Klausen MK, Thomsen M, Wortwein G, et al: The role of glucagon-like peptide 1 (GLP-1) in addictive disorders. Br J Pharmacol 179(4):625–641, 2022 34532853

Lerman C, Schnoll RA, Hawk LW Jr, et al: Use of the nicotine metabolite ratio as a genetically informed biomarker of response to nicotine patch or varenicline for smoking cessation: a randomised, double-blind placebo-controlled trial. Lancet Respir Med 3(2):131–138, 2015 25588294

Lindson N, Chepkin SC, Ye W, et al: Different doses, durations and modes of delivery of nicotine replacement therapy for smoking cessation. Cochrane Database Syst Rev 4(4):CD013308, 2019a 30997928

Lindson N, Klemperer E, Hong B, et al: Smoking reduction interventions for smoking cessation. Cochrane Database Syst Rev 9(9):CD013183, 2019b 31565800

Lindson-Hawley N, Banting M, West R, et al: Gradual versus abrupt smoking cessation: a randomized, controlled noninferiority trial. Ann Intern Med 164(9):585–592, 2016

McClure EA, Baker NL, Hood CO, et al: Cannabis and alcohol co-use in a smoking cessation pharmacotherapy trial for adolescents and emerging adults. Nicotine Tob Res 22(8):1374–1382, 2020 31612956

Moore D, Aveyard P, Connock M, et al: Effectiveness and safety of nicotine replacement therapy assisted reduction to stop smoking: systematic review and meta-analysis. BMJ 338:b1024, 2009 19342408

Oliveira P, Ribeiro J, Donato H, et al: Smoking and antidepressants pharmacokinetics: a systematic review. Ann Gen Psychiatry 16:17, 2017 28286537

Oon-Arom A, Likhitsathain S, Srisurapanont M: Efficacy and acceptability of varenicline for alcoholism: a systematic review and meta-analysis of randomized-controlled trials. Drug Alcohol Depend 205:107631, 2019 31678838

Park ER, Chang Y, Quinn V, et al: The association of depressive, anxiety, and stress symptoms and postpartum relapse to smoking: a longitudinal study. Nicotine Tob Res 11(6):707–714, 2009 19436040

Patnode CD, Henderson JT, Melnikow J, et al: Interventions for Tobacco Cessation in Adults, Including Pregnant Women: An Evidence Update for the U.S. Preventive Services Task Force. Rockville, MD, Agency for Healthcare Research and Quality, 2021

Prochaska JJ, Gill P, Hall SM: Treatment of tobacco use in an inpatient psychiatric setting. Psychiatr Serv 55(11):1265–1270, 2004 15534015

Rigotti NA, Benowitz NL, Prochaska J, et al: Cytisinicline for smoking cessation: a randomized clinical trial. JAMA 330(2):152–160, 2023 37432430

Rose JE, Behm FM: Combination treatment with varenicline and bupropion in an adaptive smoking cessation paradigm. Am J Psychiatry 171(11):1199–1205, 2014 24934962

Schwartz J, Fadahunsi O, Hingorani R, et al: Use of varenicline in smokeless tobacco cessation: a systematic review and meta-analysis. Nicotine Tob Res 18(1):10–16, 2016 25646351

Siegel SD, Lerman C, Flitter A, et al: The use of the nicotine metabolite ratio as a biomarker to personalize smoking cessation treatment: current evidence and future directions. Cancer Prev Res (Phila) 13(3):261–272, 2020 32132120

Slemmer JE, Martin BR, Damaj MI: Bupropion is a nicotinic antagonist. J Pharmacol Exp Ther 295(1):321–327, 2000

Steinberg MB, Greenhaus S, Schmelzer AC, et al: Triple-combination pharmacotherapy for medically ill smokers: a randomized trial. Ann Intern Med 150(7):447–454, 2009 19349630

Thomas KH, Martin RM, Knipe DW, et al: Risk of neuropsychiatric adverse events associated with varenicline: systematic review and meta-analysis. BMJ 350:h1109, 2015 25767129

U.S. Department of Health and Human Services: Smoking Cessation: A Report of the Surgeon General. Atlanta, GA, U.S. Department of Health and Human Services, Centers for Disease Control and Prevention, National Center for Chronic Disease Prevention and Health Promotion, Office on Smoking and Health, 2020.

Vatsalya V, Gowin JL, Schwandt ML, et al: Effects of varenicline on neural correlates of alcohol salience in heavy drinkers. Int J Neuropsychopharmacol 18(12):pyv068, 2015 26209857

Walker N, Howe C, Glover M, et al: Cytisine versus nicotine for smoking cessation. N Engl J Med 371(25):2353–2362, 2014 25517706

West O, Hajek P, McRobbie H: Systematic review of the relationship between the 3-hydroxycotinine/cotinine ratio and cigarette dependence. Psychopharmacology (Berl) 218(2):313–322, 2011 21597990

Williams JM, Gandhi KK, Benowitz NL: Carbamazepine but not valproate induces CYP2A6 activity in smokers with mental illness. Cancer Epidemiol Biomarkers Prev 19(10):2582–2589, 2010 20719908

Williams JM, Anthenelli RM, Morris CD, et al: A randomized, double-blind, placebo-controlled study evaluating the safety and efficacy of varenicline for smoking cessation in patients with schizophrenia or schizoaffective disorder. J Clin Psychiatry 73(5):654–660, 2012a 22697191

Williams JM, Gandhi KK, Lu S-E, et al: Nicotine intake and smoking topography in smokers with bipolar disorder. Bipolar Disord 14(6):618–627, 2012b 22938167

Yammine L, Green CE, Kosten TR, et al: Exenatide adjunct to nicotine patch facilitates smoking cessation and may reduce post-cessation weight gain: a pilot randomized controlled trial. Nicotine Tob Res 23(10):1682–1690, 2021 33831213

Zangen A, Moshe H, Martinez D, et al: Repetitive transcranial magnetic stimulation for smoking cessation: a pivotal multicenter double-blind randomized controlled trial. World Psychiatry 20(3):397–404, 2021 34505368

Zevin S, Benowitz NL: Drug interactions with tobacco smoking: an update. Clin Pharmacokinet 36(6):425–438, 1999 10427467

Zullino DF, Delessert D, Eap CB, et al: Tobacco and cannabis smoking cessation can lead to intoxication with clozapine or olanzapine. Int Clin Psychopharmacol 17(3):141–143, 2002

8

Engaging Individuals Into Treatment

Although most adult tobacco users want to quit, only about half report trying to quit each year. Even those who report a strong desire to quit may still encounter difficulty engaging in the treatment process. Counseling approaches that include motivational components can be effective in helping people consider change or make small steps forward. Motivational interviewing (MI) is an evidence-based intervention designed to specifically engage individuals who are not ready to change, help resolve ambivalence about change, and plan initial steps toward change (Miller and Rollnick 2013). The MI approach was developed for working with individuals with substance use disorders (SUDs) and is quite different from traditional, confrontational counseling approaches. MI is considered a patient-centered approach that allows the individual to contribute to the treatment goals.

Motivational Interventions

Motivational interventions can vary in the number of sessions provided and have been adapted for a variety of uses. One meta-analysis of MI revealed weak or insufficient evidence of its effectiveness for smoking cessation (Lindson et al. 2019b), although it remains widely used in clinical practice. Other analyses have found a benefit from MI, especially in adolescent populations (Heckman et al. 2010). This conflicting evidence may be due to limitations of current clinical trials that have different methodologies, populations, settings, and therapists. The role of MI may be to encourage people to use tobacco treatment or initially try to quit, and evaluating its effect only on long-term quitting minimizes its potential impact.

The Stages of Change model of behavior change, discussed earlier in Chapter 4, provides a framework for characterizing people into groups (i.e., precontemplation, contemplation, preparation, and action) based on their readiness to change a behavior (Prochaska and DiClemente 1992). Although thought of as discrete entities, the stages are much more dynamic, and individuals may not progress through them in an orderly way. It can be important to recognize that if someone does express a desire to change, treatment should not be delayed, and motivational language and techniques can be integrated into other approaches. On the other hand, mismatches between the patient's stage of change and clinician interventions can result in disappointment and treatment dropout. Traditional smoking cessation interventions have been geared almost exclusively toward individuals in the preparation stage, although there is growing evidence that people in other stages should be encouraged to participate in treatment, with a range of other options.

If someone seems unready to immediately take steps to change, as expressed by their language or actions, motivational counseling interventions can be helpful. For example, if someone is very resistant, or even opposed, to changing their tobacco use, they may not even want to discuss it. They may feel shame about past failed attempts or be concerned that health care providers will scold them. They would very likely not want to join a "stop smoking" group that is action-oriented and focused on quitting behaviors such as setting a quit date. Rather than confronting such individuals about their possible resistance, using MI offers a more open-ended approach that is supportive and nonconfrontational. This may help the person establish trust with the therapist and better reveal their fears or concerns about changing that may have presented barriers in the past.

For people in the precontemplation or contemplation stage, the initial goal for the clinician may be to simply guide these patients to a higher stage of change. Rather than advising an immediate quit attempt, clinicians should consider helping patients move forward in the change process by providing education and feedback, exploring the pros and cons of quitting, developing rapport and trust, normalizing ambivalence about quitting, and affirming any statements indicative of motivation to quit smoking. In addition, patients should be advised that safe and effective strategies are available to assist them. Sometimes individuals may not be able to verbalize a clear message that they are ready to change although their behavior suggests that they are willing to take steps. More commonly, patients are ambivalent about quitting and feel demoralized and ashamed because of their unsuccessful past attempts to quit. Some may express a desire to quit but not feel confident that they can be successful or lack the support needed to make a successful quit attempt. Patients can be encouraged to try treatments while receiving motivational counseling, and the counseling can be focused on trying different strategies while the person is still using tobacco.

Resolving ambivalence about behavior change is a key feature of motivational counseling. Because the patient determines the goals, the approach is collaborative, nonjudgmental, and person-centered. Techniques such as expressing empathy, actively listening, reflecting on what one has heard, and building self-efficacy are at the core of MI. Clinicians also should expect that the change process may take longer and progress more slowly with those who are in earlier stages of change.

Many patients can benefit from interventions at the start of treatment that help to increase their motivation to quit using tobacco. One such intervention is providing brief personalized feedback, which is a motivator for change. Ways to do this include completing a tobacco assessment that includes information about the patient's health consequences from tobacco and their level of dependence. This can be supplemented with an exhaled carbon monoxide reading, if available. One advantage of this reading is that it provides real-time feedback about the impact of carbon monoxide and reduced blood oxygen on the cardiovascular system. Other techniques include a decisional balance exercise listing the risks and benefits of continued tobacco use versus quitting. A discussion of consequences associated with tobacco use that the person is already experiencing can be helpful in establishing the risks of continued use and relevance to the patient. A list of tobacco consequences to consider is provided in Table 8–1. In general, motivational interventions are most likely to be successful when the clinician is empathetic, promotes patient autonomy (e.g., choice among options), and avoids arguments. Interventions that also support the patient's self-efficacy, or their sense that they can be successful, are also relevant and effective in increasing motivation.

Using motivational counseling techniques is essential because individuals will progress at different rates and/or demonstrate changing motivation to quit. It will be common for some patients to relapse

Table 8–1. Consequences of tobacco use

Major health consequences	Other consequences/barriers to recovery
Premature death	Financial hardships
Heart and vascular disease	More employment difficulties
Acute and chronic lung disease	More housing difficulties
Cancers	Poorer mental health
Other chronic diseases (diabetes, peptic ulcer disease, gum disease)	More suicidal ideation, attempts
	More relapse to drugs and alcohol
Severe coronavirus disease 2019 (COVID-19) illness	Social stigma and shame
	Wrinkles and poorer appearance
	More fires in home
	Higher doses of affected psychiatric medications

during treatment, and it makes sense to have an approach that is in keeping with these real-world issues and allows for alternative goals. Those who are unready to commit to abstinence should be encouraged to stay in treatment to gain knowledge and skills that can help them in future quit attempts. MI has a large literature supporting its use across a wide variety of problem behaviors, including engaging patients in smoking cessation treatment (Lindson et al. 2019b). Many opportunities exist for good-quality MI training (https://motivationalinterviewing .org/motivational-interviewing-training).

The Spirit of Motivational Intervention

Even if MI is not conducted in the strictest sense, the "spirit" of MI is applicable for many clinical interactions and can help promote behavior change. The spirit of MI is based on three key elements: collaboration between the therapist and the patient; evoking or drawing out the patient's ideas about change; and emphasizing the patient's autonomy. This includes the use of non-stigmatizing and hopeful language and is part of an overall engagement approach. Although most tobacco users report that they want to or have been considering quitting, the thought of quitting forever can still be intimidating. A common clinical question asked is "Do you want to quit smoking (or tobacco use)?" but this may not be a truly helpful approach for several reasons. First, it is a closed-ended question that can limit discussion and stop conversation by asking for a yes or no response. Additionally, wanting to stop using tobacco is not really a yes or no question for most. Many recognize the harms or consequences they are experiencing from tobacco use, yet they may be unable or unready to change. This ambivalence related to "wanting" to quit but believing they lack the confidence, skills, or urgency to do so leaves many people feeling stuck and discouraged. Memories of prior attempts can contribute to feeling helpless and increase resistance about trying again. Further complicating this is that quitting tobacco has almost always been presented to people as "cessation." This is a poor term that undermines the concept of tobacco use as an addiction. *Cessation* refers to a specific action in a moment in time and is not a process or a continuing event like *treatment*, which is the preferred, more neutral, term.

The thought of cessation, or the abrupt and complete stopping of tobacco, can seem overwhelming to many. Certainly, if anyone wants to quit, they should be assisted without delay, but for some, the action-oriented language of this traditional approach ("quit smoking groups," "quit services") may be too directive or limiting and therefore less attractive. An alternative approach would allow tobacco users to take steps forward (even without a commitment to quitting forever), which is consistent with the clinical approach to most other chronic diseases. Twelve-step self-help programs for other addictions, such as Alcoholics Anonymous, refer to the process of quitting substances as "one day at a time" for just this reason. Using language that frames tobacco as an SUD necessitating treatment can support positive messaging that is more engaging and supportive and thus allows a more patient-centered approach. The word *treatment* underscores this as an addiction or chronic disease, reducing shame and stigma. It also implies that there are alternatives to self-help (quitting on your own, without treatment), which, unfortunately, although the least successful approach, is also the most common way people try to quit.

If immediate quitting is not the goal, a collaborative effort can be made to develop alternative goals. This is consistent with motivational approaches and may result in more engagement, or entry, into tobacco treatment. For hard-to-reach populations, changing the message to be more engaging may be essential. Again, even the use of language about "quitting" or "stopping" may feel negative to some people. Tobacco users often feel intense shame about their ongoing use and inability to quit. Conversely, they may also perceive more benefit from tobacco than is realized. Aspects of an engagement approach are shown in Table 8–2. Education about the nature of addiction and withdrawal can help reduce stigma and blame. Positive messages of empowerment, such as "tobacco independence" or "tobacco recovery," can shift the narrative to acknowledge improved quality of life when one is not dependent on substances. Tailored messaging has been shown to work and can be helpful in reaching populations with behavioral health comorbidities. Old messages of tobacco as self-medication or effective coping can be reframed into hopeful tobacco-free recovery narratives. Many people struggle to overcome the challenges associated with having a mental illness or an addiction. A positive and powerful message can be that individuals do not have to die from tobacco use, especially when they have achieved recovery in other areas. They can also work on overcoming tobacco use as another part of their recovery journey from other addicting substances. Underscoring all of this is hope and empowerment.

Establishing a therapeutic alliance is important in the treatment of all patients. Most will not realize that it usually takes several attempts to stop using tobacco and will need to be strongly encouraged to remain in treatment following an unsuccessful attempt. A positive therapeutic relationship will help them feel comfortable returning to treatment, whatever the outcome. Advice is best given in a nonjudgmental,

Table 8–2.   Key components of an engagement approach

Be empathetic, be supportive, and express hope

Provide education about tobacco use disorder and evidence-based treatments

Explore motivation using the 5R's, including repetition

Avoid using only action-oriented words such as "cessation" and "quitting" and frame the experience as treatment

Be collaborative in supporting patients to set appropriate goals

Conduct a tobacco assessment and provide personalized feedback about the impact of tobacco on health, finances, and other consequences empathetic, and supportive manner that is positive, flexible, and engaging. A sense of optimism and a clear message of hope are also important. Patients are reassured by messages that you will "stick with them" through disappointments and multiple quit attempts, if necessary. The style can be strongly supportive, motivational, and even "coach"-like to help individuals learn about the impact of tobacco, use the tobacco treatment medications effectively, and learn how to manage setbacks. Note that this may be in contrast to other messages they have received about tobacco in the past, such as that it is not the "right time" to stop or that they cannot succeed simply because they have a diagnosis of serious mental illness. Clear language about the hope of treatment and the possibility of an eventual tobacco-free life is essential.

In addition to individual counseling, groups can also incorporate motivational techniques and provide support and information to those not immediately ready to stop using tobacco. Learning About Healthy Living (LAHL) is a group treatment approach developed for working with patients with serious mental illness. This manualized group treatment intervention has become a national model for working with tobacco users in mental health settings and is a 20-session group treatment approach designed to enhance motivation to change (Williams et al. 2009).

The goals of LAHL are to raise awareness about tobacco use consequences and educate participants about the benefits of treatment. LAHL includes sessions on other wellness topics, which helps make the materials appealing to a broader audience and links tobacco use with an overall healthy lifestyle. A group format can help provide support and modeling for participants, who can benefit from seeing peers succeed and develop new coping strategies. LAHL has been well received by mental health staff and patients (Lee et al. 2011). Revised in 2024, the LAHL manual is available online as a publicly available resource (https://rwjms.rutgers.edu/sites/default/files/2024-04/2012_lahl.pdf). The 2024 edition of LAHL includes new sections on vaping, electronic cigarettes, and other aspects of harm reduction.

Doing a tobacco assessment can be a helpful initial approach with less motivated patients. This assessment not only provides information about tobacco addiction and the impact of tobacco use but is also a clinical intervention that can provide an opportunity for open-ended tobacco discussion. Many versions of tobacco assessments are available, ranging from brief to comprehensive. The LAHL treatment manual includes a brief assessment tool that can also be used as self-assessment if appropriate to the clinical setting. It includes questions about the type and amount of tobacco use (not limited to cigarettes only), questions about the person's level of dependence and motivation to change, and a brief inventory of health consequences. The assessment is not focused on prior quit attempts, which, although an essential factor for someone working on quitting, may be less relevant to someone who is guarded or just beginning to discuss this issue for the first time. This type of brief assessment also provides an opportunity for the patient to receive some personalized feedback about how tobacco may be impacting them. In this way, it is a clinical activity that can open the door to talking about tobacco.

Revisiting tobacco use at periodic intervals, especially when tobacco-caused illnesses (e.g., bronchitis) or other special situations (e.g., pregnancy, child with asthma) occur, can sometimes motivate individuals to change. Tobacco use can be integrated into other clinical discussions about health, mental health, and addictions, as well as non-health-related topics such as employment, housing, or even monthly budgeting because tobacco use negatively impacts all of these areas. Adding tobacco use into other treatment groups or counseling sessions is an efficient way to introduce the topic to larger audiences and is consistent with other wellness and recovery goals the individual may be working on.

Using the 5R's

The "5R's" refers to a motivational strategy for addressing tobacco use that emphasizes Relevance, Risks, Rewards, Roadblocks, and Repetition (Fiore 2008). Discuss with patients the Relevance of tobacco to them. Have them consider how stopping tobacco use may be relevant to their health or other goals. A personalized inventory of their tobacco use consequences may have a greater impact on changing behavior than a generic information sheet. Review the Risks of continued tobacco use, which includes not only medical diseases but financial and other consequences (reviewed in Table 8–1). Have them think about the Rewards or benefits of changing, and include specific examples of what could get better in a tobacco-free life. A discussion of current and past Roadblocks to quitting is important and could include such factors as living with someone who uses tobacco or having experienced significant withdrawal symptoms in the past. Discussing these issues encourages problem-solving or trying alternative approaches on future attempts. These techniques can be used to solidify motivation to change, reduce shame, and increase hope. Finally, Repetition is essential because it will likely take several discussions to help people consider change as well as several attempts to successfully achieve their goals.

Co-Occurring Disorders

The coexistence of a mental illness and an SUD is common and known as a co-occurring disorder. This comorbidity is known to complicate diagnosis and treatment, and integrated care that addresses both is recommended. Co-occurring disorders are associated with worse outcomes on many measures, including symptom severity, service utilization and hospitalization, suicidality, and homelessness. With co-occurring disorders, patients may not express a desire for complete abstinence from substances or may struggle to navigate complex health care systems. New approaches for working with patients with co-occurring disorders emerged in the 1990s and emphasized integrated care models that were supportive and motivational. Integrated treatment, ideally provided by a single clinical team, helps prevent patients from getting lost or excluded and provides a unified approach for recovery.

Tobacco use disorder (TUD) is an addiction and should be viewed as a co-occurring disorder in behavioral health settings, on par with other SUDs. Applying models for other co-occurring disorders to tobacco is a useful and practical clinical approach. Co-occurring approaches for addressing tobacco use can have a long-term perspective that includes motivational interventions to enhance change and lessen resistance. This emphasis on inclusion and engagement is key because most people have already tried to stop using tobacco in the past and may remember it as a negative experience. Approaching tobacco use as a wellness issue or an addiction, rather than as a lifestyle choice or a shameful practice, enhances the collaborative relationship and de-emphasizes "quitting" as the only viable outcome.

Principles of co-occurring disorders treatment are a helpful guide to integrating tobacco treatment into other clinical services and are reviewed in Table 8–3. Effective strategies such as MI, use of psychopharmacology, and inclusion of support services (e.g., case management and housing programs) can be applied to the treatment of TUD. A treatment team approach allows everyone to reinforce the message of the benefits of a tobacco-free lifestyle and may reduce clinician burnout. Although treatment for co-occurring disorders works, change can come slowly, and having a long-term perspective is helpful (Drake et al. 2005). Incorporating tobacco treatment into other treatments for mental

Table 8–3. Using the co-occurring disorders model to work with lower motivated tobacco users

For co-occurring mental health and substance use disorders	For co-occurring tobacco use
Provide integrated mental health and addiction services; parallel or sequential services are less effective than integrated services	Offer tobacco assessment and treatment services in the behavioral health setting, rather than refer people out
Provide comprehensive services	Include a range of services from assessment to treatment, including options for those at different stages of change, and evidence-based approaches for counseling and medication
Provide treatments matched to motivational level because not everyone will have abstinence from substances as an initial goal	Consider intervention for all tobacco users, including an education/ motivational approach for those not immediately ready to make changes
Take a long-term treatment perspective because patients with co-occurring disorders are highly prone to relapse even after full remission	Have appropriate expectations because not all patients will be ready to stop using tobacco immediately; use repetition and allow time for change
Conduct continuous assessment of substance use, especially if it seems that treatment is not working	Reassess to ensure key aspects are not being ignored, such as other tobacco use, factors contributing to craving and relapse, role of mood, or other symptoms
Use motivational interventions as a way to promote engagement in treatment, and be supportive of alternative points of view	Use open-ended questions, reflective listening, and other techniques to help address ambivalence and tip the balance toward eventual change
Use psychopharmacology to reduce mental illness symptoms, reduce withdrawal and craving from substances, and improve outcomes	Consider medications, which can reduce craving and withdrawal and lead to successful smoking reductions as well as subsequent quitting, even in those who do not seem immediately ready to change

Table 8–3. Using the co-occurring disorders model to work with lower motivated tobacco users (*continued*)

For co-occurring mental health and substance use disorders	For co-occurring tobacco use
Include services such as case management to provide outreach and support in the community	Encourage support services staff to reinforce the message of a tobacco-free lifestyle and to not assist patients in purchasing or obtaining tobacco
Include supported housing in the services	Consider factors associated with more quitting behavior, such as not living with a tobacco user or having restrictions on tobacco use in the home (e.g., smoking allowed outdoors only)

Note. Many approaches for co-occurring disorders can be adapted and utilized for tobacco users.

illness or SUDs offers many opportunities to intervene and underscores it as an important part of overall recovery.

Opt-Out Tobacco Treatment

Strategies for tobacco intervention in clinical settings have traditionally been reactive, in terms of responding to a patient's stated desire to quit. This model provides treatment typically to the person who is motivated to try to stop and willing to take the next steps, and it is quite different from what is done for other chronic diseases, where the provider recommends the optimal treatment plan regardless of, and without overtly considering, the person's motivational state. For other chronic diseases, it is assumed that the person wants to have better health, and the benefits of treatment are known and the next steps are taken automatically. In a clinic, for example, everyone has their heart, blood pressure, and other vital signs assessed automatically and without additional verbal consent. With regard to tobacco, however, practice has been much more cautious, suggesting that providers can only proceed with further discussion if the patient verbally agrees and expresses interest in trying to quit. This approach greatly limits access to treatment for many tobacco users who may be ambivalent or unable to quickly express the complex ways they feel about quitting. For example, someone may feel very interested in wanting to quit, yet not be immediately ready or lack confidence that this is something they can achieve. Motivation to quit is not really a simple yes or no answer, but it has been used in the past to direct next steps for only a small subset of tobacco users.

As an attempt to deliver tobacco interventions more routinely and reach more individuals, "opt-out" practices have emerged in medical settings. This model of service delivery suggests that the health care team provide consistent and systematic intervention to all tobacco users, not just those who are motivated to try to quit (Richter and Ellerbeck 2015). These interventions can range from routine administration of nicotine replacement therapy (NRT) and counseling to warm handoffs initiating proactive calls to quitlines or tobacco treatment clinics. Individuals may refuse or "opt out" of this at any time, but studies find that only about 15% of tobacco users generally do (Nahhas et al. 2017). Opt-out approaches have been associated with greater enrollment in services, greater use of tobacco treatment medications, and higher abstinence rates in people receiving these services compared with those not receiving them (Buchanan et al. 2017; Nahhas et al. 2017). Proactive tobacco strategies are also effective for people with behavioral health conditions (Japuntich et al. 2020).

Although SUD treatment is more effective for those with motivation to change, it can also be effective in some who are not motivated for abstinence. For example, mandated or compulsory treatment can be effective for alcohol and other drug use disorders (National Institute on Drug Abuse 2012), and tobacco-free policies enhance smoking cessation. Additionally, many other chronic diseases have a strong behavioral component to them, including diet and weight management for hypertension, non-insulin-dependent diabetes mellitus, and others. Treatment is provided to individuals with diagnosed conditions regardless of their stated motivation to change or their desire to try behavioral approaches. This includes providing medications to individuals with these conditions, such as type 2 diabetes, even if they are unwilling or unable to comply with any behavior changes, such as diet.

Other SUDs are often addressed with greater urgency in the clinical setting than tobacco. If, for example, an individual is found to have a cocaine use disorder, this will generate a series of interventions, including detailed assessments, SUD counseling treatment services, and aftercare referrals, without the clinician typically asking the person if they want them. Although this is not "forced" treatment in the strictest sense, ambivalence is common in people with SUDs, and they may be fearful about acknowledging the need for change. A directive approach sends the hopeful message that the person has value and would benefit from treatment. The same standards should apply to tobacco treatment, where everyone gets the benefit of a quality intervention every time. This approach can be delivered as a system-wide initiative that strives to reach every tobacco user and is consistent with other health care service delivery.

Smoking Reduction

Smoking reduction has been debated in the past as a viable treatment strategy because of concerns about giving conflicting messages to patients about ongoing tobacco use. Even small amounts of smoke exposure are toxic and cause harm, but encouraging individuals only to lessen their tobacco intake could create a false sense of security and take attention away from the ultimate goal of quitting. There is no safe established amount of smoke exposure, and even secondhand smoke (i.e., environmental) exposure can cause cancer and heart disease. However, recent evidence shows that if individuals are able to reduce their cigarette intake significantly (by 50% or more), they reduce their level of dependence over time, which in turn increases their chances of subsequently quitting. Quantifying smoking reduction with biomarkers such as exhaled carbon monoxide level can be more reliable than measures of cigarettes per day.

Using medications during tobacco reduction further increases the chances of a meaningful reduction in tobacco use and subsequent quitting (Lindson et al. 2019a). There is less evidence to support the use of behavioral interventions alone (without medication) for smoking reduction. All tobacco users should be encouraged to use pharmacotherapy because it can be effective even in individuals who are not immediately ready to stop smoking. Reduction without medication can be difficult and result in significant tobacco withdrawal symptoms. Use of medication by patients willing to try to reduce their smoking can help in several ways by limiting withdrawal and craving and blocking some of the pleasurable effects of smoking. Use of NRT is associated with significant reductions in smoking, as well as an increased likelihood of quitting smoking in populations unable or unwilling to quit (Lindson-Hawley et al. 2016). Varenicline is also effective for smoking reduction. A large trial of varenicline versus placebo for 24 weeks in people not willing or able to immediately quit smoking demonstrated that the use of varenicline was associated with much higher rates of abstinence from smoking at 6 months and 12 months (Ebbert et al. 2015). In this study, individuals given varenicline (or placebo) were encouraged to reduce smoking by 50% within the first 4 weeks and then again by 50% in the next 4 weeks, with the goal of reaching complete abstinence by 12 weeks. Varenicline reduction strategies have been so successful that they are part of the FDA-approved label for usage recommendations. Treatments for people not yet ready to quit smoking but willing to reduce their cigarette consumption are viable strategies.

Case Example

Pat is 50 years old and smokes 20 cigarettes per day. When discussing smoking, she says, "I'd like to quit but I think deep down inside that I'll never be able to. I just enjoy smoking too much." Without prompting, Pat explains that she does not smoke out in public because she is embarrassed. She says she stays inside a lot to smoke. When asked if she has health problems, she describes having gum problems and losing her teeth in addition to getting frequent respiratory illnesses. When asked how much it costs her to smoke, Pat says it costs $7 a day. The interviewer provides feedback that this is about $50 a week, $200 a month, and $2,500 a year. Pat says this surprises her, that she didn't think about the total cost, and if she stopped smoking, she would use the money to buy more things for her son and family. She says she feels guilty spending all her money on cigarettes. She describes feeling bound to the cigarette, "like it's running my life," and disappointed that she has been unable to quit in the past. She also experienced significant withdrawal symptoms during past attempts, such as irritability, that caused her to relapse.

What Are the Concerns in This Case?

This is a common clinical scenario in which MI can be helpful. If the interviewer were to stop at only the first comment, "I just enjoy smoking too much," assuming that nothing can be done because the patient is getting too much enjoyment from cigarettes, an opportunity is lost. Initially, Pat seems very discouraged, like she has given up on trying to quit smoking. Without much prompting, however, she quickly reveals many consequences that she is experiencing from cigarettes. She seems to be in the contemplation stage because she acknowledges that she would like to quit but does not have any immediate plans to try. She also fears being unsuccessful again and does not feel confident in her ability to quit. The interviewer can listen to her in a supportive way, without telling her that she should quit, and ask open-ended questions such as, "Can you tell me about any health problems you have had from smoking?" or "How much does it cost to smoke?" As Pat discusses her experiences, she reveals the many ways in which she does not enjoy smoking and it is a problem for her. Thinking about the pros and cons of continuing to smoke is part of a decisional balance exercise that helps Pat build the argument to consider change. Acknowledging her frustration and disappointment about not being able to quit in the past conveys a message of support and can strengthen the therapeutic alliance.

Key Points

- Every tobacco user should receive treatment of some kind, with an emphasis on engaging people in strategies to change.
- Motivational approaches should encourage collaboration between the therapist and the patient, evoke the patient's ideas about change, and emphasize the patient's autonomy.
- Smoking reduction can be a viable approach and is more successful with the use of pharmacotherapy that reduces tobacco withdrawal and blocks some of the pleasurable effects of smoking.
- Opt-out strategies for tobacco use are being employed increasingly in clinical settings and result in greater engagement with and use of tobacco treatments.

References

Buchanan C, Nahhas GJ, Guille C, et al: Tobacco use prevalence and outcomes among perinatal patients assessed through an "opt-out" cessation and follow-up clinical program. Matern Child Health J 21(9):1790–1797, 2017 28702864

Drake RE, Wallach MA, McGovern MP: Future directions in preventing relapse to substance abuse among clients with severe mental illnesses. Psychiatr Serv 56(10):1297–1302, 2005

Ebbert JO, Hughes JR, West RJ, et al: Effect of varenicline on smoking cessation through smoking reduction: a randomized clinical trial. JAMA 313(7):687–694, 2015 25688780

Fiore M: Treating Tobacco Use and Dependence: 2008 Update. Washington, DC, U.S. Department of Health and Human Services, 2008

Heckman CJ, Egleston BL, Hofmann MT: Efficacy of motivational interviewing for smoking cessation: a systematic review and meta-analysis. Tob Control 19(5):410–416, 2010 20675688

Japuntich SJ, Hammett PJ, Rogers ES, et al: Effectiveness of proactive tobacco cessation treatment outreach among smokers with serious mental illness. Nicotine Tob Res 22(9):1433–1438, 2020 31957794

Lee JGL, Ranney LM, Goldstein AO, et al: Successful implementation of a wellness and tobacco cessation curriculum in psychosocial rehabilitation clubhouses. BMC Public Health 11:702, 2011 21917179

Lindson N, Klemperer E, Hong B, et al: Smoking reduction interventions for smoking cessation. Cochrane Database Syst Rev 9(9):CD013183, 2019a 31565800

Lindson N, Thompson TP, Ferrey A, et al: Motivational interviewing for smoking cessation. Cochrane Database Syst Rev 7(7):CD006936, 2019b 31425622

Lindson-Hawley N, Banting M, West R, et al: Gradual versus abrupt smoking cessation: a randomized, controlled noninferiority trial. Ann Intern Med 164(9):585–592, 2016 26975007

Miller WR, Rollnick S: Motivational Interviewing, 3rd Edition. New York, Guilford, 2013

Nahhas GJ, Wilson D, Talbot V, et al: Feasibility of implementing a hospital-based "opt-out" tobacco-cessation service. Nicotine Tob Res 19(8):937–943, 2017 27928052

National Institute on Drug Abuse: Principles of Drug Addiction Treatment, 3rd Edition. NIH Publication No 12-4180. Bethesda, MD, National Institute on Drug Abuse, December 2012

Prochaska JO, DiClemente CC: Stages of change in the modification of problem behaviors. Prog Behav Modif 28:183–218, 1992 1620663

Richter KP, Ellerbeck EF: It's time to change the default for tobacco treatment. Addiction 110(3):381–386, 2015 25323093

Williams JM, Ziedonis DM, Vreeland B, et al: A wellness approach to addressing tobacco in mental health settings: Learning About Healthy Living. Am J Psychiatr Rehabil 12(4):352–369, 2009

9

Preventing a Return to Smoking and Creating a Tobacco-Free Lifestyle

Sustaining any type of behavior change is challenging and associated with high rates of relapse. Indeed, substance use disorders (SUDs) are best viewed as chronic diseases associated with a long-term relapsing and remitting course. Although a lot of emphasis is put on initial quitting, most people relapse within the first 7 days, making relapse prevention a critical part of eventual success. In SUDs, relapse is typically described as the first return to substance use after an initial period of abstinence, although it is often helpful to distinguish between a lapse and a relapse. A *lapse*, or slip, is a single unplanned use of alcohol or drugs. *Relapse* happens when a recovery plan is completely abandoned and the person has returned to patterns of baseline or repeated use. It may also be defined as a return to substance use lasting 7 days or longer. Underscoring all of this are experiences of craving and withdrawal that undermine attempts for abstinence and influence lapses and relapses. Learning theories suggest that lapses and relapses are also linked to past settings or situations associated with substance use. Availability of the substance and use of alcohol or other substances are also factors that can lead to lapse and relapse. Helping patients avoid or overcome these scenarios is essential because even a single episode of post-quit smoking ("lapsing") can lead to relapse.

Most people lapse and engage in some smoking during the first 7 days after quitting, and the experience of acute tobacco withdrawal symptoms is a likely contributor. Tobacco withdrawal includes symptoms of irritable or depressed mood, trouble sleeping, feeling frustrated, difficulty concentrating, restlessness, or feeling hungry. Educating patients about the nature and duration of tobacco withdrawal symptoms helps them understand that these are temporary symptoms that will get better during the first few weeks of abstinence and can be relieved in large part by tobacco treatment medications. Psychosocial approaches may even further lessen symptoms of withdrawal, providing education and support around coping and optimizing the use of medications. For example, continuing to wear nicotine patches after smoking lapses promotes recovery of abstinence at subsequent outcomes (Ferguson et al. 2012).

Newer models conceptualize relapse not as a single event but as a more dynamic process related to the integration of many possible factors. Stress is a known factor linked to relapse. The neural circuits involved in stress overlap substantially with the brain systems involved in drug reward. Chronic substance use contributes to an enhanced stress system caused by dysregulation of the hypothalamic-pituitary-adrenal (HPA) axis and alterations in brain reward and emotional systems. This implies that individuals with addiction experience enhanced vulnerability to all types of stressors in addition to an altered response to stress. This sensitivity, or heightened state of stress, is present not only during acute withdrawal but also for longer periods lasting months or longer. Protracted abstinence syndromes are physiological mood changes that can persist for months after the individual has completed the acute phase of substance withdrawal. Symptoms can include irritability, persistent sleep disturbances, and tremor. Treatment was often limited in the past to reassurance and education because many or all of these symptoms are expected to resolve spontaneously over time. This approach was often inadequate; protracted abstinence symptoms contribute to significant distress and can lead to substance relapse. The role of maintenance medication treatment beyond the acute withdrawal phase has increased because this has been proven to reduce the risk for relapse, at least in part, by lessening protracted abstinence symptoms for alcohol, tobacco, and opioids.

Craving is an elusive concept that is portrayed as a defining characteristic of addiction. Although it has a complex relationship to relapse, high craving is generally reported more by people with higher levels of nicotine dependence (Germovsek et al. 2021). Craving is common among people who smoke, even during periods of typical smoking, and can fluctuate throughout the day and be influenced by smoking cues as well as the time since last tobacco use. Measurement of craving can be momentary or last a longer period of time (e.g., 24 hours). It is generally worse after abstinence and can persist for months or longer after a successful quit. Differences in methodology for how craving is assessed may explain some inconsistencies in research findings. Post-quit craving may be more indicative of withdrawal and therefore more linked to outcome, although most studies fail to specifically test whether craving influences outcomes in quitting smoking (Wray et al. 2013). Still, addressing craving is universally included in clinical interventions (medications and counseling) for addictions treatment.

Negative reinforcement theory suggests that a strong motivator in seeking and using substances is the desire to alleviate bad or negative feelings or experiences (also called *negative affect*). Substance withdrawal is an example of negative reinforcement that contributes to relapse; other examples include negative moods associated with depression, stress, or other mental illness. The ability to overcome or persist despite distress is associated with better outcomes and less relapse. The need to deliberately control one's actions and behaviors when quitting smoking can lead to fatigue and result in craving and relapse. A related idea, *delay discounting*, refers to how people devalue or discount the long-term benefits of quitting and instead choose the immediate reward of smoking. Higher delay discounting is also associated with more relapse and decreased activity in the prefrontal cortex, making this a potential area of interest for studies of relapse prevention. Although discussed as single entities in the research literature, these conceptual models likely interact to contribute to lapse and relapse in individuals. New research suggests that anhedonia may also be a unique symptom of tobacco withdrawal that is more pronounced in people who are more heavily dependent on smoking (Cook et al. 2017).

Although most studies evaluate short-term outcomes for quitting, such as the first 3–6 months when the risk for relapse is greatest, some individuals relapse at later time points. It is estimated that as many as 10% relapse even after 1 year of abstinence. This risk (10% relapse per year) continues for subsequent years (Hughes et al. 2008), making the need to practice relapse prevention skills a long-term endeavor. Relapse prevention efforts should also be adaptable to accommodate different needs over time.

These conceptual models form the basis for specific strategies to prevent relapse. Effective strategies include pharmacological treatment, behavioral approaches, or combinations of both. One challenge when interpreting relapse prevention studies is that they often differ in methods, and not every study shows a benefit. Some extended treatments may include all people who smoke, not just those who were initially successful in quitting. Many of these treatments have favorable results and work by retaining "lapsers" in treatment and having them recommit to abstinence. In practice, each patient who uses tobacco requires personalized treatment, and clinical judgment may support extended treatment with medications and counseling, even in the absence of conclusive evidence. Fewer of these studies exist because studies with long follow-up periods or longer durations of treatments are inherently more difficult and more expensive to complete.

Relapse Prevention Counseling

Relapse prevention counseling (RP counseling) is an evidence-based practice based in cognitive-behavioral therapy (CBT). It is a method of teaching and practicing healthy behaviors and skills through learning, and the emphasis is on enhancing self-control strategies. In RP counseling, coping strategies are individualized and based on the specific types of problems encountered by an individual and their usual coping styles. This type of counseling can be integrated into other approaches and can be delivered via individual, group, or self-help formats.

In the treatment setting, discussion of relapse does not have to begin only after the quit attempt. It often makes sense to assess and review prior barriers to quitting during assessment or the initial steps of treatment. This is called conducting a *relapse analysis* and includes a detailed discussion of both the positive and negative aspects of prior quit attempts. Clinicians should ask about methods used, such as support, counseling, or medications, including whether they were used at an adequate dosage and for a long enough time. Most people try to quit on their own, without the benefit of behavioral counseling or medications, and a review of how that may have undermined prior attempts can reinforce the need for treatment going forward. In addition to reviewing the use of evidence-based treatment approaches, the relapse analysis can include individual factors that may have contributed to relapse during prior attempts. It is also important to reinforce positive steps taken or examples of tobacco-free coping. Often, the individual feels shame about prior relapse and may frame the discussion negatively, such as "I only quit for 2 weeks." Numerous attempts are often needed for sustained success, and practicing quitting for any period should be supported positively. The emphasis can be on lessons learned and ways to enhance future attempts to avoid common pitfalls.

Most standard treatments include six to eight sessions of counseling, but ongoing booster sessions of RP counseling may be helpful to some. Sessions generally become less frequent over time, although some patients may benefit from prolonged contact and ongoing support. Tobacco treatments lasting longer than 12 weeks, in general, are better than briefer approaches, although the best evidence for prevention of smoking relapse is associated with extended-duration medications or use of self-help materials (Murray et al. 2022). Patients are taught in RP counseling that they have an opportunity to learn from past behaviors and to use that information to promote improved abstinence.

A plan for increasing support outside of the treatment setting is essential to preventing relapse. Anything that supports the tobacco-free effort or makes it harder to use tobacco can be employed. Ways to obtain support include being in tobacco-free spaces or consulting with tobacco-free individuals. Spending time in the many types of tobacco-free public spaces such as libraries, theaters, restaurants, or parks can be helpful and can reinforce goals for tobacco-free recreation and lifestyles. Tobacco-free rules in the household and negative attitudes about tobacco use from family members enhance outcomes and contribute to greater success in quitting. Conversely, continued tobacco use in the home by anyone can be a sizable barrier to success. Having identified support persons helps patients during a challenging period and supplements efforts in the clinical setting. These individuals can be non-tobacco-using family members or friends, or peers with similar lived experience. Supported housing staff, case managers, and other support services can be very helpful to individuals with behavioral health conditions who are living in the community. The availability of online support or smartphone applications provides another option. Often, these applications are free and have the advantage of being available at any time of day or night; they can also provide links to support emails or connections with online groups in which people provide mutual self-help support. Building a larger nonsmoking network over time helps prevent relapse and reinforces the continued commitment to abstinence.

Celebrating quitting is an important concept to discuss explicitly with patients. This minimizes feelings of loss around tobacco and emphasizes the many positive ways quitting improves health and quality of life. Addiction is a disease in which one gives up everything to continue doing one thing—use substances. Recovery is the opposite of addiction and can be conceptualized as giving up one thing (the continued use of substances) to gain and continue everything else that is good in life. Reminders of the benefits are important when challenges emerge. Building in alternative rewards during the quitting process is essential and should be highly individualized. Some patients might choose to spend the money saved from tobacco on alternative, healthier pleasures or to save for a specific, larger goal such as a vacation. Scheduling or structuring time to do pleasant tobacco-free activities can make quitting seem less onerous and lead to other benefits such as enhanced mood or greater support. In the clinical setting, celebrating quitting can be done by acknowledging a patient's achievements in a group setting or by awarding certificates or other recognition.

Helping patients recognize high-risk states or situations that lead to tobacco use and subsequently avoid or overcome them is the major focus of RP counseling. Numerous factors, including social support and self-efficacy, account for some general vulnerability to relapse. When high-risk situations are encountered, these factors, along with current mood state and the degree to which effective coping behaviors are performed, can determine whether relapse occurs. Specifically, RP counseling helps individuals in three ways. The first is helping them recognize situations in which they feel at higher risk to use tobacco. These are often referred to as *triggers* and can include external (e.g., people, places, things) and internal (e.g., mood states, feelings) states or situations that the person associates with smoking. Common triggers are reviewed in Table 9–1. RP counseling also helps patients identify high-risk situations and explores the concept of tobacco craving.

External events include being around other tobacco users, being in places or situations where the patient used tobacco previously, and encountering tobacco-related paraphernalia. For example, buying groceries at a store where tobacco was also purchased may cause intense feelings of wanting to smoke that can only be avoided by going to an alternative store. Having any tobacco in the home during a quit attempt should be discouraged because the easy availability will be difficult to overcome for most and lead to intense cravings or urges to use. Similarly, seeing others using tobacco often leads to temptation, lapse, or relapse. Even the smell of tobacco smoke that can linger on fabrics or surfaces can be enough to trigger craving and relapse. This is why health care professionals should always be discouraged from using tobacco at work because they may be inadvertently affecting craving in others.

Table 9–1. Relapse prevention techniques to combat cues and triggers

Relapse prevention counseling (RP counseling) is an evidence-based practice based in cognitive-behavioral therapy. RP counseling is a method of teaching and practicing healthy behaviors and skills through learning, and the emphasis is on enhancing self-control strategies. Coping strategies are individualized and based on the specific types of problems encountered by an individual and their usual coping styles. RP counseling can be integrated into other approaches and can be delivered via individual, group, or self-help formats for craving triggers: people, places, things, and mood states.

People	Explain to patients that it is not necessary to become socially isolated when quitting smoking, but that it is important to stay away from people who use tobacco, offer cigarettes, or smell of tobacco as much as possible. When avoidance is impossible or impractical, encourage patients to make others aware of their quit attempt and to ask them not to offer more cigarettes in the future.
Places	Places can serve as triggers for smoking, particularly places where a lot of smoking is happening or that especially remind the person of smoking. People with serious mental illness who live in a group home or participate in a day program usually have access to places dedicated to smoking. It will be important for these patients to avoid such places and to plan other locations where they can socialize with people who do not smoke. An effective strategy for people in day treatment settings, where smoke breaks are common, may be to ask what other non-smoking patients do between groups.
Things	Patients should remove/avoid any objects or paraphernalia associated with smoking, including lighters, matches, ashtrays, cigarette packs, coffee, alcohol, and street drugs. Check to make sure that the patient has discarded all paraphernalia and has removed cigarette butts and old packs from their environment.

Table 9–1.	Relapse prevention techniques to combat cues and triggers (*continued*)
Mood states	Quitting smoking can create feelings of sadness, discouragement, and anxiety. Patients can expect to get less pleasure out of activities for a week or more; those who succeed in quitting smoking learn to tolerate these withdrawal-related negative feelings until they disappear. Many people use smoking to manage unpleasant feelings and boredom, so learning other ways to manage these negative mood states is one of the most important skills someone can learn when quitting. Offer to help patients cope with triggers throughout the course of treatment.
Other addictions	Other compulsive behaviors or addictions can trigger cravings for smoking, including alcohol, marijuana, cocaine, and other substances. Compulsive behaviors such as overeating and overspending, sexual activity, and gambling can also be triggers.

Internal states that can lead to relapse include boredom, negative moods, anger, urges to use, and intoxication with other substances. Increasingly, these negative emotional states, such as emotional pain, malaise, and dysphoria, are understood as directly related to relapse and the persistence of addiction. In this way, using drugs as a form of self-medication to alleviate suffering or distress, termed *negative reinforcement*, helps explain the compulsive nature of addiction and substance-seeking even in the context of severe life consequences. Overcoming internal states can be challenging because simply avoiding these types of triggers is often not possible. Therapies to cope with and manage mood states can be effective, as can medications. People with serious mental illness may find themselves in additional or unique situations or develop symptoms that contribute to smoking relapse, including boredom or symptoms of depression or anxiety. Weekends or other periods of unstructured time can also contribute to relapse. Use of other substances, such as alcohol or cannabis, can increase craving for tobacco and impact behavioral factors, such as impulsivity, that contribute to relapse.

Once recognized, the next steps involve being able to avoid or more effectively cope with the situations, feelings, and behaviors associated with tobacco use. Removing triggers, including paraphernalia, from the environment can be an important step when preparing for a quit date that helps to reduce relapse later. This includes not only tobacco but also lighters, ashtrays, and other reminders of tobacco use. In addition to avoiding tobacco products, it may be helpful to avoid other people using tobacco, at least temporarily; if this includes family, friends, and others in the household, a plan for coping with this challenge is necessary. Significant others can be encouraged to smoke outdoors or not directly in front of the patient. Sometimes it makes sense to include such people in the quit plan and to get their commitment to support their loved one's efforts and not entice them inadvertently. Avoiding places where tobacco is used can include places in and around the home as well as in the community. Patients in behavioral health treatment often remark that the culture of smoking at the clinic or shared residence adds to the challenge of remaining abstinent. Having patients create a list of "safe" tobacco-free spaces can be helpful in planning for new patterns of behavior, help avoid boredom, and support a tobacco-free lifestyle.

Developing coping skills is essential because not all cues and triggers can be avoided, and encountering some is inevitable and perhaps critical to long-term success. This includes helping patients identify their feelings and surroundings, manage them, and learn and practice alternative skills. Coping with cues and triggers may include many types of strategies that can be highly individualized. One example is practicing relaxation, such as a deep breathing exercise. Another idea might be referring to a mantra or to a short list of reasons why the person wants to stay quit. Some may find it helpful to reach out to a support person or peer to talk about their experience. Distraction can be helpful to shift the focus of attention to another activity. Almost anything can be used for distraction, including practicing hobbies, watching television or movies, reading, or going out, making this process very patient-driven. Brainstorming possible ideas and scenarios ahead of time can be helpful as someone prepares to quit. This can be a good time for them to try a new hobby or activity because they may have extra money saved from not buying tobacco. Over time, as patients confront different situations successfully without smoking, some urges will lessen and even go away.

Talking about tobacco withdrawal and craving is an important part of RP counseling. Cravings can continue to occur for weeks or months after quitting and are not a sign that the patient is not serious about quitting. When a person tries to quit, they have strong urges or could be exposed to cues that remind them of tobacco even when they feel determined to quit, and for this reason, it is important to anticipate these cues and triggers and to develop and practice new coping skills. Cravings are normal, and people experience them differently. They often have a time-limited duration, and one strategy can be to try to "ride out" or "surf" this urge as cravings approach, peak in intensity, and then fade. Having a list of specific options that the person could try in the context of craving could help them feel more empowered and prepared. Different strategies might be helpful in different situations, and thus having more than one approach seems practical.

Although the goal is for someone not to smoke at all starting with the quit date, lapses and relapses inevitably will occur. Patients should be supported in a nonjudgmental way when reporting these lapses to reduce shame and disappointment and prevent treatment dropout. A supportive, problem-solving approach can result in discussion of an immediate plan of action (which may include revised strategies) and a commitment to continued treatment. Whenever possible, the goal is to try to prevent a lapse from becoming a relapse.

If the patient has relapsed back to smoking, discuss the details of what has happened. Patients may believe they have failed or disappointed you and may be concerned that you will even be angry with them. Reassure them that your role is to be encouraging and support-ive and is not contingent on them quitting. Remind them that you are pleased that they attended the session to discuss their difficulties and concerns. Some patients may only phone to tell you that they are drop-ping out and fail to come in. A no-show for an appointment can imply that the patient has been using tobacco and is feeling disappointed and ashamed. Quick response to these calls is needed and will encour-age them to come in for an appointment to discuss things. Even if the patient feels ambivalent about a goal of abstinence, they should be encouraged to remain in treatment and attend sessions to learn and prepare for future attempts.

In the context of a lapse or relapse, it can be important to give posi-tive feedback and support and to validate any steps the patient has taken toward quitting. Individuals can be rewarded for taking steps such as using nicotine replacement therapy (NRT), having a reduced carbon monoxide reading, or even for expressing motivation or resolve. Empathize with any frustration expressed about having failed to quit. Determine whether there are any barriers to quitting that can be eas-ily resolved, and whether these barriers are largely due to low moti-vation to quit, low self-confidence, or lack of knowledge. Try to elicit specific obstacles during the discussion. Inquire specifically whether the patient purchased tobacco and if they are currently carrying it with them, because having the substance available will make it harder to abstain from use. If a patient is using NRT, they should be encouraged to carry some short-acting gum or lozenge with them to use as needed for withdrawal and craving. This idea of using short-acting NRT as a rescue medication should be encouraged and can be discussed and modeled in group settings.

RP counseling can include a variety of practical and problem-solving strategies. It may be necessary to increase the intensity of treatment and assistance after a lapse or relapse. It is fundamental to individual-ize what to do next according to the symptoms and distress experi-enced by the patient. This might include increasing the intensity and frequency of cessation counseling or medications (discussed in more detail later in the sections "Medications for Preventing Relapse" and "Extended Counseling for Preventing Relapse"). It may be important to review the specific directions or dosing of medications because patients commonly underdose NRT and may be using medications in a suboptimal way. A medication change might be considered if the patient experienced side effects or was not using one of the first-line strategies (varenicline or combination NRT).

When lapses and relapses occur, it is essential to encourage the person to stay in treatment. If they feel unready to consider a new quit attempt, stress that they will still benefit from treatment through continued support and learning about the benefits of quitting and consequences of smoking. Patients can feel hopeful that they are sticking with treatment and learning things that can help them with future attempts. Discussing the consequences of tobacco use that the patient is specifically experiencing can be helpful for enhancing motivation to change. This includes not only health consequences but financial and quality-of-life issues as well. A menu of topics can be considered for discussion, such as reviewing the pros and cons of quitting in a decisional balance exercise. The 5R's (discussed also in Chapter 8) can be repeated to enhance motivation to take steps forward; this motivational strategy emphasizes the Relevance of tobacco to the person, the Risks of continued tobacco use, the Rewards or benefits of changing, current or past Roadblocks to quitting, and Repetition because it will likely take several discussions to help people consider change and successfully achieve their goals. When possible, clinicians should focus on those aspects that are most clearly relevant to the patient.

After a relapse, the clinician should assess the need for and barriers to tobacco treatment medication use, in particular if withdrawal symptoms contributed to the patient's slip or relapse. They should reassess the patient's readiness to return to abstinence or work on enhancing motivation for a future attempt. Patients will benefit from their clinician recognizing the progress they had made, even if they have slipped or relapsed. The patient and the clinician should then discuss what was learned with this quit attempt and when the patient would like to think about trying again. The clinician should express their ongoing commitment to work with the patient and to help them eventually quit smoking.

Follow-up telephone calls are another way to deliver RP counseling and support. These can be done to continue abstinence after a tobacco-free inpatient hospitalization. In the hospital setting, abstinence is forced, and typical environmental cues have been removed. Patients may feel more motivated, especially if their illness is tobacco-related. Brief counseling support and medication can be provided in the hospital. A nurse or health care provider trained in tobacco treatment can offer proactive follow-up calls and a plan for continued tobacco treatment medications. Generally, this post-hospitalization follow-up can last for several weeks and be supplemented with written materials.

Although RP counseling interventions are often delivered in group or individual sessions, they also can be delivered via self-help booklets that individuals read on their own (Agboola et al. 2010; Brandon et al. 2007). This strategy may be particularly helpful for subgroups such as postpartum females or people who are heavily dependent on smoking (Brandon et al. 2012; Unrod et al. 2016). It can also provide an easy-to-use resource to individuals who may have quit on their own without the benefit of counseling treatment. A series of 10 RP booklets plus 9 additional pamphlets on increasing social support, mailed to patients over the course of 18 months, was effective at reducing relapse in several studies (Brandon et al. 2016; Simmons et al. 2018). The pamphlets are based in CBT and traditional relapse prevention but are presented as brief recovery narratives that help personalize the material. The booklets emphasize the health and other benefits of long-term tobacco abstinence, stress and mood management, anticipation of potential high-risk situations, and the use of coping responses. These Forever Free self-help booklets are available free through the Moffitt Cancer Center, where they were developed, and they have also been translated into Spanish (see Table 9–2 for booklet topics and a link to access). Given that this intervention is freely available, it could have great public health impact if employed more widely.

Mindfulness and contingency management are two other behavioral strategies that have been studied to prevent relapse. Mindfulness-based treatments target the emotional dysregulation associated with substance use and may be most effective when combined with evidence-based strategies. In contrast to traditional RP counseling, which employs distraction and avoidance of aversive emotional experiences, mindfulness approaches emphasize acceptance. This includes paying attention nonjudgmentally to things in the present moment. Data show that mindfulness approaches can reduce symptoms and improve emotion regulation difficulties, but evidence for a long-term benefit for relapse prevention is currently lacking (Sancho et al. 2018).

Medications for Preventing Relapse

The ongoing use of tobacco treatment medications can be individualized, but most people should be encouraged to continue them for a duration of 6 months. Nicotine withdrawal symptoms are generally the

Table 9–2. Forever Free self-help booklets

Booklet topics

Booklet 1: An Overview

Booklet 2: Smoking Urges

Booklet 3: Smoking and Weight

Booklet 4: What If You Have a Cigarette?

Booklet 5: Your Health

Booklet 6: Stress and Mood

Booklet 7: Lifestyle Balance

Booklet 8: Life Without Cigarettes

Booklet 9: Benefits of Quitting Smoking

Booklet 10: The Road Ahead

Source. https://moffitt.org/research-science/research-teams/tobacco-research-and
-intervention-program-trip/trip-research/forever-free-self-help.

most severe in the first week after quitting, although they can continue for weeks or longer. Over time, although their intensity may be reduced, they can still undermine success and contribute to relapse. Studies of medications taken for less than 6 months show greater relapse, and some people may want to continue their medication for much longer periods. A meta-analysis of 81 studies of behavioral and pharmacological relapse prevention techniques found that the strongest effect was for extended medications, particularly varenicline (Livingstone-Banks et al. 2019), but extended bupropion, NRT, or a combination of NRT and bupropion can be helpful as well (Agboola et al. 2010; Coleman et al. 2010). The mixed evidence of a long-term benefit from NRT could be the result of less adherence with the medication over time (Schnoll et al. 2015), but having the option to use NRT as needed as a rescue medication for intermittent craving or high-risk situations offers advantages. Extended treatment with nicotine replacement may help prevent relapse by reducing cravings (Germovsek et al. 2021).

Two studies have evaluated the benefit of continued varenicline in participants who were successful in an aided quit attempt (using varenicline and counseling). Those randomly assigned to continue varenicline after a successful quit at 12 weeks were about 2.5 times more likely to stay abstinent at 6 months compared with those given placebo. This effect was maintained through the 1-year follow-up period. A second study enrolled people with serious mental illness (schizophrenia or bipolar disorder) in a similar design. Successful quitters at 12 weeks were randomly assigned to continue varenicline (or placebo) for another 40 weeks. Despite ongoing CBT sessions, relapse back to smoking was rapid during the first 4 weeks of placebo treatment (weeks 12–16) but was much attenuated in the varenicline continuation group (Evins et al. 2014). At week 52, 60% of the varenicline group was still abstinent, versus 19% of the placebo group. This study has importance for helping people with serious mental illness who need longer-term and more intensive treatments to successfully quit smoking. At study end (52 weeks), when medication was stopped, relapse rates were high, supporting an even longer possible role for medication continuation. This type of maintenance medication for prevention of relapse is the standard of care for opioid use disorder and has been used increasingly in other SUDs as well.

Extended Counseling for Preventing Relapse

There have been a few studies of extended counseling and medications in people who were initially successful in quitting smoking for 8–12 weeks. These studies examined bupropion, NRT, or nortriptyline in combination with extended counseling (Hall et al. 2004, 2009, 2011). Two studies have shown the benefit of extended CBT in people who quit smoking with an initial 12-week treatment (Hall et al. 2009, 2011). The extended treatment options were typically 11 additional sessions over 40 weeks, bringing the full duration of treatment to 1 year. The counseling conditions generally produced a more robust effect than the medications, and the additional costs to provide this counseling were considered nominal and cost-effective (Barnett et al. 2014).

Case Example

Alex is an English professor who wants to stop smoking. He has been successful in reducing his cigarette consumption from 20 per day to 7 or 8 per day but experiences intense cravings that make it difficult to quit completely and cause him to relapse. He has made several past attempts during which he quit for 3–6 months. During these times, he used nicotine medications for short periods, such as a nicotine patch for 4 weeks. Alex also has a history of alcohol use disorder, although he stopped using alcohol completely 5 years ago. He attended some mutual self-help groups for the first year of abstinence and is confident in his ability to continue abstaining from alcohol. In the past year he started taking a selective serotonin reuptake inhibitor (SSRI) that has been very helpful in reducing his chronic symptoms of excess anxiety and worrying. He knows he has used cigarettes in the past as a way to cope with anxiety symptoms and stress. Now he has started dating someone who does not smoke and who supports him quitting.

What Are the Concerns in This Case?

Although this patient is motivated to stop, his efforts have been undermined by frequent relapses back to smoking caused by numerous factors. A thorough interview can help to identify the cues, triggers, and moods that make him vulnerable to relapse. Alex has many strengths that can help him be successful. He is motivated and understands the risks of continued tobacco use. He has been successful in quitting other substances and wants to develop healthier ways of coping with stress. His partner does not smoke and supports him quitting. He should be applauded for trying again, and it can be helpful to reframe these attempts as practice that informs future quitting rather than as failures.

Alex has some experience with nicotine replacement but has not used it optimally. Using combination NRT (patch plus short-acting lozenge or gum) or using it for a longer period of time (up to 6 months) may help reduce the risk for relapse. Short-acting formulations can be helpful throughout the day to overcome intermittent cravings, and the patient can be encouraged to always carry them with him. He can also use behavioral strategies to overcome urges, such as reaching out to a support person, practicing relaxation, or using distraction to focus on another activity. He enjoys writing and can think about journaling or spending more time on his other hobbies. Accepting feelings and allowing them to pass over him (like a wave) can help him deal with not only urges to smoke but also feelings of anxiety. It would be worthwhile to discuss what strategies helped him when faced with an alcohol craving in the past and whether these could help him overcome tobacco use as well. He could consider using 12-step techniques or attending groups he may have found helpful in the past. He should try to avoid buying or keeping tobacco or related paraphernalia, such as ashtrays, because this will increase temptation.

Key Points

- Relapse prevention counseling is a method of practicing healthy behaviors and skills that is individualized to the specific types of problems encountered by an individual.
- Helping patients recognize high-risk states or situations that lead to tobacco use and subsequently avoid or overcome them is the major focus of counseling.
- Although relapse prevention counseling interventions are often delivered in group or individual counseling sessions, they can be delivered effectively through self-help booklets that individuals read on their own.
- The use of tobacco treatment medications for at least 6 months' duration should be encouraged to reduce the risk of relapse.

References

Agboola S, McNeill A, Coleman T, et al: A systematic review of the effectiveness of smoking relapse prevention interventions for abstinent smokers. Addiction 105(8):1362–1380, 2010 20653619

Barnett PG, Wong W, Jeffers A, et al: Cost-effectiveness of extended cessation treatment for older smokers. Addiction 109(2):314–322, 2014 24329972

Brandon TH, Vidrine JI, Litvin EB: Relapse and relapse prevention. Annu Rev Clin Psychol 3:257–284, 2007 17716056

Brandon TH, Simmons VN, Meade CD, et al: Self-help booklets for preventing postpartum smoking relapse: a randomized trial. Am J Public Health 102(11):2109–2115, 2012 22994170

Brandon TH, Simmons VN, Sutton SK, et al: Extended self-help for smoking cessation: a randomized controlled trial. Am J Prev Med 51(1):54–62, 2016 26868284

Coleman T, Agboola S, Leonardi-Bee J, et al: Relapse prevention in UK Stop Smoking Services: current practice, systematic reviews of effectiveness and cost-effectiveness analysis (iii–iv). Health Technol Assess 14(49):1–152, iii–iv, 2010 21040645

Cook JW, Lanza ST, Chu W, et al: Anhedonia: its dynamic relations with craving, negative affect, and treatment during a quit smoking attempt. Nicotine Tob Res 19(6):703–709, 2017 28486709

Evins AE, Cather C, Pratt SA, et al: Maintenance treatment with varenicline for smoking cessation in patients with schizophrenia and bipolar disorder: a randomized clinical trial. JAMA 311(2):145–154, 2014 24399553

Ferguson SG, Gitchell JG, Shiffman S: Continuing to wear nicotine patches after smoking lapses promotes recovery of abstinence. Addiction 107(7):1349–1353, 2012 22276996

Germovsek E, Hansson A, Karlsson MO, et al: A time-to-event model relating integrated craving to risk of smoking relapse across different nicotine replacement therapy formulations. Clin Pharmacol Ther 109(2):416–423, 2021 32734606

Hall SM, Humfleet GL, Reus VI, et al: Extended nortriptyline and psychological treatment for cigarette smoking. Am J Psychiatry 161(11):2100–2107, 2004 15514412

Hall SM, Humfleet GL, Muñoz RF, et al: Extended treatment of older cigarette smokers. Addiction 104(6):1043–1052, 2009 19392908

Hall SM, Humfleet GL, Muñoz RF, et al: Using extended cognitive behavioral treatment and medication to treat dependent smokers. Am J Public Health 101(12):2349–2356, 2011 21653904

Hughes JR, Peters EN, Naud S: Relapse to smoking after 1 year of abstinence: a meta-analysis. Addict Behav 33(12):1516–1520, 2008 18706769

Livingstone-Banks J, Norris E, Hartmann-Boyce J, et al: Relapse prevention interventions for smoking cessation. Cochrane Database Syst Rev 2019(10):CD003999, 2019 31684681

Murray RL, Zhang Y-Q, Ross S, et al: Extended duration treatment of tobacco dependence: a systematic review and meta-analysis. Ann Am Thorac Soc 19(8):1390–1403, 2022 35254966

Sancho M, De Gracia M, Rodríguez RC, et al: Mindfulness-based interventions for the treatment of substance and behavioral addictions: a systematic review. Front Psychiatry 9:95, 2018 29651257

Schnoll RA, Goelz PM, Veluz-Wilkins A, et al: Long-term nicotine replacement therapy: a randomized clinical trial. JAMA Intern Med 175(4):504–511, 2015 25705872

Simmons VN, Sutton SK, Meltzer LR, et al: Long-term outcomes from a self-help smoking cessation randomized controlled trial. Psychol Addict Behav 32(7):710–714, 2018 30284878

Unrod M, Simmons VN, Sutton SK, et al: Relapse-prevention booklets as an adjunct to a tobacco quitline: a randomized controlled effectiveness trial. Nicotine Tob Res 18(3):298–305, 2016 25847293

Wray JM, Gass JC, Tiffany ST: A systematic review of the relationships between craving and smoking cessation. Nicotine Tob Res 15(7):1167–1182, 2013 23291636

10

Approach to Tobacco in the Clinical Setting

Need for Systems Change in Health Care Settings

In addition to the clinical interventions delivered by individual health care providers, changes can be made at the systems level to implement more widespread or systematic change. Systems changes can be local, such as implementing standardized tobacco practices in a clinic or hospital, or widespread and far-reaching, such as regional or national tobacco policies that affect sales or clean indoor air.

Systematic interventions for screening and intervention for tobacco use are necessary to allow everyone on the health care team to assist at every opportunity. Promoting health systems change has proven effective in reducing the number of people using tobacco (Centers for Disease Control and Prevention 2014). Health systems change involves institutionalizing prevention and treatment interventions in health care settings and integrating these into routine clinical care. Implementation strategies can include 1) systems for routine tobacco screening and treatment; 2) widespread support for staff education on evidence-based practices; and 3) policies that restrict tobacco in the environment and support the provision of tobacco services. Clinical reminders can be implemented through an electronic medical record (EMR). Rates of tobacco intervention (such as with 2A's and an R; see "Implementing

Screening and Brief Intervention" section) can be evaluated and tracked as a quality improvement initiative. Setting benchmarks or goals for the practice and providing feedback to staff at regular intervals may be a useful part of any strategy. Overriding all of this is a need for strong and clear leadership. Administration needs to articulate the vision and provide ongoing support for those implementing change. It is helpful to increase buy-in for addressing tobacco because it is often a low-priority issue, particularly when systems are already stressed or understaffed. These strategies are discussed in more detail in the discussion that follows and are shown in Table 10–1.

Implementing Screening and Brief Intervention

Every patient contact can include a brief tobacco intervention, such as asking about tobacco use. Ask, Advise, and Refer (2A's and an R) is an evidence-based strategy that can be done in less than 3 minutes' time. All patients should be screened for tobacco use at regular intervals, and this should include questions about all types of tobacco products, including electronic cigarettes. Clearly defined processes for documenting assessments can also ensure that they are completed routinely, at every visit, or repeated at least every 6 months. All staff can be trained to deliver brief interventions that include referral if they are unable to provide further treatment. Even a few minutes of feedback and counseling can be effective in motivating behavior change and have a later impact that may not be evident in the current moment. Processes to refer or link individuals with more comprehensive services should be standardized. Referral can be within the same practice or clinic, if other staff members are available to provide services, or to an outside treatment, such as a telephone quitline or a specialized clinic, provider, or group. The 2A's and an R model is an abbreviated version of the 5A's (Ask, Advise, Assess, Assist, and Arrange Follow-Up) that recognizes the constraints that may prevent some health care practices from delivering intensive tobacco treatment services and thus provides a minimum of screening, brief intervention, and referral. This model of service delivery was developed to address substance use problems in emergency settings and has been shown to be useful in a variety of health care practices (U.S. Department of Health and Human Services 2020).

Table 10–1. Examples of health care systems changes that support treatment for tobacco use disorder

---

Implement screening and brief intervention

Implement proactive (opt-out) strategies to reach every tobacco user

Designate specific staff to provide intensive tobacco treatments and support their professional development as a Certified Tobacco Treatment Specialist (CTTS)

Change the environment of care to de-normalize tobacco use

Develop alternative activities to smoke breaks, including recreation or meditation options

Develop and implement tobacco-free treatment grounds

Restrict staff smoking and offer treatment resources

Conduct recurring assessments that include a minimum of information about tobacco use severity and readiness to change

Develop and implement policies that define standards for treatment and responsible staff

Include tobacco in policies and practices for other substance use disorder treatments or wellness/recovery initiatives

Provide withdrawal management interventions for all tobacco users during periods of temporary abstinence

Support staff with training resources and supervision

Develop peer-led support groups or activities led by former tobacco users

---

Proactive Strategies (Opt-Out)

Strategies for tobacco intervention in clinical settings have traditionally been reactive in terms of responding to a patient's stated desire to quit. Implementing a newer opt-out system of tobacco treatment is another way to address systems change.

The opt-out model of service delivery suggests that the health care team provide consistent and systematic intervention to all tobacco users, not just those who are motivated to try to quit (Richter and Ellerbeck 2015). This can include a range of interventions from routine administration of nicotine replacement therapy (NRT) and counseling to proactive calls or "warm handoffs" to quitlines or tobacco treatment

clinics. Individuals may refuse or "opt out" of this at any time, but studies find that only about 15% of tobacco users generally do (Nahhas et al.
2017). These approaches have been associated with greater enrollment
in services, greater use of tobacco treatment medications, and higher
abstinence rates than are seen with those not receiving these routine
services (Buchanan et al. 2017; Nahhas et al. 2017). Opt-out models are
discussed further in Chapter 8.

Designated Staff

Although everyone on the health care team can participate in
interventions for screening, brief intervention, and referral, it is helpful
to also have designated staff who provide more intensive tobacco
treatment interventions. These staff can provide either group or
individual intensive counseling, which is defined as anything more than
four sessions, lasting 10 minutes each. These counseling and supportive
services can be delivered in person or remotely via telehealth visits.
This can help the medical or prescribing team to maximize efforts by
coordinating services with a designated counselor. This counselor can
also provide education to other staff about the impact of tobacco use
on the population and the need for intervention. Specialty training
and certification as a Certified Tobacco Treatment Specialist (CTTS) is
available through the American Heart Association (www.heart.org/
en/professional/quality-improvement/healthcare-certification/cpaha
/tobacco-treatment-certification) and the Association for Addiction
Professionals (NAADAC; www.naadac.org). Similarly, specialty clinics
for tobacco treatment services have emerged, although access is still
often limited. In real-world settings, tobacco treatment specialists are
effective at providing access to more intensive treatments than the
typical health care team (Burke et al. 2015; Burns et al. 2023; McEwen et
al. 2006; Sheffer et al. 2021).

The Problem and Promise
of Behavioral Health
Treatment Settings

In the United States alone, more than 3.5 million individuals received
outpatient services in 2020 in a specialty behavioral health treatment
setting (Substance Abuse and Mental Health Services Administration

2020). At least 30%–40% of individuals with mental illness are estimated to use tobacco, which provides a tremendous opportunity to provide clinical intervention to this vulnerable group. Efforts to treat tobacco use disorder (TUD) are well suited to the behavioral health care setting because these providers have training and experience in treating other addictions. They are also trained in motivational and other effective counseling approaches, generally have more time to spend during clinical encounters, and can offer detailed assessments and access to a treatment team. Integrated models for treatment of other co-occurring (mental health and addictions) disorders are optimal and yield the best outcomes; it makes good clinical sense to extend this to the treatment of TUD.

Despite almost 30 years of recommendations to treat tobacco in the specialty behavioral health setting, even recent national data indicate that these systems still provide low levels of tobacco screening and intervention. In 2016, less than 50% of U.S. mental health treatment facilities screened patients for tobacco use, and rates of treatment intervention were lower still (Marynak et al. 2018). As of 2020, only 55% of mental health treatment facilities had smoke-free treatment environments, which is lower than general medical hospitals (92%) (Substance Abuse and Mental Health Services Administration 2020). Rates of tobacco screening and treatment are similarly low in substance abuse treatment facilities. A national survey of more than 500 outpatient substance abuse treatment programs showed that less than half (41%) offered smoking cessation counseling or pharmacotherapy (Friedmann et al. 2008). Although some progress has been made, the culture of smoking, which includes ongoing debate about rights and choices among individuals with behavioral health conditions, remains a sizable barrier (Lawn and Campion 2013).

Decades of evidence have shown that psychiatrists provide less tobacco intervention and screening than other physicians and are less familiar with relevant clinical practice guidelines (Tong et al. 2010; Young et al. 2023). This can come from a lack of education on TUD as well as negative attitudes and beliefs. Buy-in from behavioral health staff is inconsistent, and surveys show that tobacco use is often rated as a low priority (Ratschen et al. 2009; Richter et al. 2012; Williams et al. 2015). In fact, staff in behavioral health settings may exhibit greater resistance to tobacco-free policies than patients (Hehir et al. 2013; Lawn and Pols 2005) and may underestimate the motivational level of patients. Tobacco-using staff also do less to intervene with patients than non-users (Guydish et al. 2022).

Understanding the attitudes of practitioners is important because more favorable attitudes are associated with higher rates of delivering tobacco treatment (Meredith et al. 2005). Out-of-date attitudes, such as that smoking helps to reduce symptoms or that quitting worsens mental health, slow progress. Programs may worry about reduced referral rates and program income if the facility considers going tobacco-free. The worry that patients will not access treatment is particularly strong among substance use disorder (SUD) treatment centers, where private, for-profit facilities are least likely to have tobacco-free grounds (Shi and Cummins 2015; Substance Abuse and Mental Health Services Administration 2013). This suggests a coercive aspect of allowing ongoing tobacco use and some form of institutional "profiting" in these settings. Many of these concerns are not borne out in studies evaluating the impact of tobacco-free environments that show no reduction in admissions (Scheeres et al. 2020; Shi and Cummins 2015), and increasingly it is being recognized that quitting tobacco is part of recovery from a mental illness or SUD. Quitting smoking will not hinder progress and might be beneficial in ways beyond health improvement, such as reduced depression or anxiety and enhanced sobriety. A successful intervention should identify local barriers and resistance and work to identify strategies to overcome them.

Models for Systems Change Interventions for Addressing Tobacco

Addressing tobacco use in mental health and addiction treatment settings is a comprehensive effort that not only affects the delivery of new clinical treatments but also includes broader efforts to change the environment of care and to rethink policies that may have enabled tobacco use previously. Systems change initiatives can include many specific activities such as scheduling staff training or implementing new treatments or policies. These broader systems changes can have numerous benefits and help patients and staff to de-normalize tobacco use and rethink the risks and benefits of using tobacco in a way that may tip the balance toward change. Making systems change efforts also promotes people quitting tobacco because they can make it harder to use tobacco while increasing the availability of treatment services, which thus increases the overall demand for these services. Program changes can occur at all levels of care (e.g., outpatient, inpatient, residential) and can be implemented sequentially as part of an institutional change plan with specific goals, deadlines, and dedicated staff. The changes may be limited or expansive, ranging from brief, or easier, steps to more comprehensive ones that provide a variety of treatment services and place limits on staff and patient tobacco use. A program might consider the ultimate step of creating an entirely tobacco-free treatment environment that reinforces the message of health and hope to everyone and prioritizes wellness.

Several models now exist for the recommended steps for addressing tobacco in a behavioral health program. One of the first models was developed in New Jersey by John Slade, M.D., and colleagues in the 1990s. Focusing on helping addictions programs address tobacco use, he developed a "12-step" model for organizational change (Hoffman and Slade 1993) that has since been adapted and used by many other groups in mental health and addictions settings. Variations of this model were used, and shown to be successful, for implementation of statewide tobacco-free policy initiatives in substance abuse services (Brown et al. 2012; Williams et al. 2005). Updated versions include an emphasis on creating an institutional treatment plan to identify the tasks and actions required to move the program forward as well as a greater emphasis on sustainability (see, e.g., https://nyctcttac.org/wp-content/uploads/2022/05/NYC-TCTTAC-Steps-for-Addressing-Tobacco-in-your-Program.pdf). Addressing sustainability may include efforts to evaluate the plan, monitor compliance, and provide feedback to those implementing change to ensure that the initial effort does not degrade over time and is maintained as part of usual practice.

It may be helpful to conduct a program self-assessment as a first step to determine what may already be in place for addressing tobacco. The Tobacco Integration Self-Evaluation Tool (TiSET) is a 20-item scale covering six dimensions of addressing tobacco use within a behavioral health treatment program (Covell et al. 2022). Completion of the self-assessment generates a report that summarizes both strengths and areas for improvement across the dimensions of Policy and Administration, Environment, Screening/Assessment, Treatment, Staff, and Training. This report can be used to develop an institutional treatment plan that identifies priorities and includes goals, objectives, interventions, responsible persons, and projected target dates. Completion of the TiSET can be repeated to demonstrate changes within an organization or program over time. This resource and associated supporting documents can be found on the website for the Tobacco Cessation Training and Technical Assistance Center (TCTTAC) Program in New York City[1] (https://nyctcttac.org).

In order to provide comprehensive care, processes should be defined for specific clinical practices. At a minimum, this should include screening, brief intervention, and referral. Upon a positive screen for tobacco use, patients should receive a thorough assessment that attends to the severity of their TUD, as well as their willingness/readiness to change and history of prior attempts. Documentation of TUD should be included on relevant problem lists, treatment plans, and aftercare plans. Treatment planning in the behavioral health setting should always include tobacco use and does not need to be oriented only around quitting. It can include many possible interventions, such as strategies for those not immediately ready or wanting to stop that include discussion of medication and counseling options. Shared decision-making with the patient can identify measurable short- and long-term goals. Alternative goals for those not immediately interested in quitting can include learning more about tobacco use consequences or the benefits of a harm reduction approach. Minimizing the uncomfortable symptoms of tobacco withdrawal during periods of temporary abstinence can also be included as a goal. Including tobacco use in the treatment plan is consistent with other practices for treating co-occurring mental health and addictions problems and sends a message that this is an important issue.

TUD is an addiction and should be viewed and addressed as a co-occurring disorder in behavioral health settings. The principles of treatment for co-occurring disorders are a helpful guide when integrating tobacco treatment into other clinical services. The Substance Abuse and Mental Health Services Administration and other organizations support this "alcohol, tobacco, and other drugs" (ATOD) approach to behavioral health care that explicitly includes tobacco. Tobacco treatment should be offered at the same location as the mental health or addictions treatment and matched to motivational level. Patients may not express a desire for complete abstinence from tobacco as their goal, so programs can take a long-term treatment perspective and use motivational interventions to enhance change and lessen resistance. Words such as "cessation" and "quitting" should be de-emphasized because this action-oriented language is only relevant for people preparing to

---

1 NYC TCTTAC was funded by the New York City Department of Health and Mental Hygiene, through a contract with Public Health Solutions.

make a change and may be off-putting to others or sound overwhelming. An emphasis on inclusion and engagement is key because most individuals have already tried to stop using tobacco in the past and may remember it as a negative experience. Approaching tobacco as a wellness issue or an addiction rather than as a lifestyle choice or shameful practice enhances the collaborative relationship.

Effective strategies for treating co-occurring disorders that include motivational interviewing, use of psychopharmacology, and inclusion of support services such as case management and housing programs can be applied to the treatment of TUD. A treatment team approach allows everyone to reinforce the message of the benefits of a tobacco-free lifestyle. Although treatment for co-occurring disorders works, change can come slowly, so programs need to take a long-term perspective for addressing tobacco use.

Policies That Restrict Tobacco in the Environment and Support Treatment Planning

Changing policy is one of the most highly effective ways of reducing tobacco use and the harms associated with tobacco exposure. Policies are a highly cost-effective strategy that helps fewer young people to start, and more adults to quit, using tobacco. They are typically thought of in terms of defining the environment to restrict tobacco use (i.e., as smoke-free or tobacco-free), but they can also be used to set the standards of care and to shape expected practices in the clinical setting. They also help change the existing norms around tobacco in the environment. Tobacco-free policies, although challenging for some settings, are the most restrictive and most powerful intervention to eliminate tobacco and related paraphernalia from the environment and physical space. Even if a tobacco-free treatment environment is not an immediate goal, many other kinds of policy changes can be implemented to denormalize the use of tobacco, encourage tobacco users to want to quit, and increase access to treatment. Examples of other policy changes are listed in Table 10–2.

There are many examples of policies that can be used to define the expectations for tobacco treatment and treatment planning. An organization can define the minimum standards for screening and documentation practices. This can include the processes for assessment, such

---

Table 10–2. Other policy change options (alternatives to tobacco-free treatment grounds)

Prohibit staff from using tobacco alongside or in view of patients

Eliminate any practice that provides tobacco products for free or purchase

Create standing (or suggested) orders for tobacco treatment medications

Require assessment and treatment of tobacco use at all levels of care, including discharge planning and aftercare

Provide easy access to nicotine replacement products during periods of temporary abstinence

Do not require participation in tobacco counseling in order to access medications

Change substance use policies to an "alcohol, tobacco, and other drugs" (ATOD) orientation to explicitly include tobacco with other substances

Allow only non-tobacco-using staff with a minimum of 6 months' recovery from tobacco to provide tobacco treatment to patients

Replace smoke breaks with healthy (and possibly indoor) activity breaks

---

as the use of standardized assessments and timing of interventions. Policies can define the staff responsible for providing screening, counseling, or prescriptions. The organization can delineate expected interventions to reduce withdrawal symptoms when patients are subjected to periods of temporary abstinence. Standing orders for NRT and other tobacco treatment medications can be written in hospital settings to reduce barriers and facilitate care. Tobacco language can be explicitly included in other relevant policies that the organization may have around addressing wellness or other SUD or co-occurring disorders.

Making information visible in the environment of care is another way to address tobacco and to inform patients. This can include messages that reinforce the dangers of tobacco use and the availability of staff to help. New policies should be clearly communicated to patients through educational materials and signs. Additional resources such as brochures or posters can supplement treatment activities and will also educate the population served. Materials adapted for behavioral health populations may be the most suitable. Include multiple perspectives (e.g., leadership, supervisors, direct care staff, people you serve) when selecting or developing educational materials and signs. Examples of sample posters and educational materials can be found on the website for the TCTTAC (https://nyctcttac.org).

Having tobacco-free grounds at behavioral health treatment programs facilitates the greatest change in de-normalizing tobacco use by changing the environment of care and supporting tobacco treatment. "Tobacco-free grounds" refers to policies that restrict all types of tobacco use not only indoors, in buildings, but also in all outdoor areas on the grounds. Typically, these policies apply not only to patients but also to staff and visitors to the facility. Quitting tobacco is difficult in a treatment setting that allows tobacco use because of the abundance of triggers in the environment. Large regional or statewide tobacco-free policies in substance abuse treatment programs have resulted in more tobacco-related training among staff, more use of NRT and other treatments, and more positive staff beliefs toward and delivery of tobacco cessation services to patients (Brown et al. 2012; Campbell et al. 2022; Williams et al. 2005). A meta-analysis of studies of people who experienced temporary abstinence from smoking due to a stay in a tobacco-free setting (including prison, acute [medical or psychiatric] hospital, or substance abuse treatment program) showed that some participants continued abstinence after discharge (Shoesmith et al. 2021). Allowing tobacco use on campus contradicts the primary treatment mission of recovery and a drug-free lifestyle that many programs support. When tobacco use is permitted in behavioral health treatment settings, it may cause some patients to relapse back to smoking after quitting or cause others to experience smoking for the first time. Implementing policy changes that restrict tobacco use must always be accompanied by efforts to increase access to treatment and minimize tobacco withdrawal.

Providing safe and comfortable access to substance detoxification is critical in any treatment setting, even if patients choose to use tobacco after discharge. Experiencing tobacco withdrawal is uncomfortable and could negatively impact care or contribute to earlier discharges from treatment. Policies around providing medications to minimize tobacco withdrawal allow individuals to experience even brief periods of being tobacco-free, which can increase hope and motivate them in the future. Several studies show that a brief inpatient tobacco intervention that includes motivational interviewing and access to NRT results in sustained quitting following discharge (Brown et al. 2021; Metse et al. 2017; Prochaska et al. 2014).

Tobacco-free policies are intended to create a healthy environment for everyone who comes to a health care setting to receive care, visit someone, or work. Psychiatric hospitals that have undergone these changes indicate improved patient health, cleaner environment and hospital grounds, increased staff satisfaction, and more time available to provide treatment (Hehir et al. 2013). They also report fewer behavioral problems and no increase in violence after tobacco-free policies take effect, which contradicts the typical staff fear of negative effects (Riad-Allen et al. 2017; Scheeres et al. 2020; Voci et al. 2010). A permissive attitude toward tobacco use, such as "let them smoke," sends the negative message that people are not worth the effort and undermines efforts at quitting. Seemingly compassionate "smoke breaks" reinforce negative concepts such as using drugs to cope or relax. Exempting behavioral health treatment facilities from tobacco-free laws and policies aimed at protecting the public also has the potential to worsen health inequalities for people with mental illness and further their stigmatization (Williams 2008).

Supporting Staff

It is important to build up a critical mass of staff who feel equipped and confident to treat TUD. Everyone on the treatment team should contribute to supporting the patient in becoming tobacco-free. Encouraging everyone to integrate tobacco into the language and practice of other existing treatment services can maximize efforts and enhance sustainability. Clinical staff need supervision and support from administrators to implement new treatment initiatives. Prescribers need to provide access to evidence-based medications. Nonclinical staff support staff and peer counselors can enhance and extend the efforts of treatment providers. Former tobacco users can model healthy behaviors. It may be helpful to delineate roles for different members of the treatment team and to establish guidelines for expected knowledge, skills, competencies, and resources for training. A helpful tool for implementing staff tobacco guidelines has been developed by the TCTTAC (https:// nyctcttac.org/wp-content/uploads/2022/04/NYC-TCTTAC-Roles-in -Implementing-Tobacco-Treatment-for-all-Staff.pdf).

Changing behavioral health care systems to address tobacco use requires leadership and administrative support. These efforts are not trivial and can take months to years to successfully implement and sustain. Such changes can only succeed with administrative support and buy-in from the entire organization. Leadership plays a pivotal role in shaping the overall mission and creating an environment that energizes others for change. Having a designated champion is associated with success and sustained effort in organizational change in other areas of health care. Leadership also sets the tone for raising the priority of addressing tobacco use and can be helpful when roadblocks and barriers arise. In addition to supporting policy initiatives, leadership should ensure that staff receive adequate training and supervision to be successful in their roles and measure and track outcomes to demonstrate the success of these efforts over time.

Providing recovery assistance to staff who use tobacco will help the program be successful regardless of whether the decision is made to be entirely tobacco-free. Staff members who smoke are common in behavioral health treatment centers (Bernstein and Stoduto 1999; Guydish et al. 2022; Hahn et al. 1999). Staff can be held to a higher no-tobacco-use standard (compared with patients) that also helps them attain better health. This should always be done in a compassionate and nonpunitive way that provides staff who use tobacco with support and assistance, including making resources available such as free NRT or allowing them to use work time to call a quitline or access other tobacco treatment services. Helping tobacco-using staff is an important consideration because studies show that health professionals who use tobacco provide fewer cessation services and rate their ability to help patients as lower than their non-tobacco-using colleagues (Braun et al. 2004; Guydish et al. 2022; Slater et al. 2006). They also have more negative attitudes about the impact of smoke-free environment policies (Hehir et al. 2013). Other restrictions on staff smoking are an important part of an overall policy addressing tobacco use in facilities, even if there is no plan to be entirely tobacco-free. Examples can include not allowing staff to smoke alongside patients, because reinforcing substance-using behavior is often contrary to the organizational treatment philosophy.

Training is a necessary component of an overall approach to systems change. Many behavioral health providers lack knowledge about evidence-based practices for treating TUD, and access to education is limited. Not one behavioral health practice was included in a comprehensive review (381 studies) on the impact of training health care professionals about tobacco (Carson et al. 2012). Education models have been developed that are effective and well received by behavioral health audiences (Ratschen et al. 2009; Williams et al. 2015, 2019). Despite low levels of knowledge, behavioral health staff support educational efforts and believe this is part of their role. Interventions aimed at training health professionals can be an important first step in increasing the delivery of tobacco treatments. Staff attitudes improve with education and support, and behavioral health staff provide more tobacco treatments after receiving an intensive training experience that addresses buy-in (Williams et al. 2015, 2019).

Peers, Family, and Support Services

Numerous other influences on tobacco use exist in the community and outside of the health care system. Community-based initiatives are helpful in transforming the social norms around the way tobacco is promoted and used and support the broader treatment effort. This community includes family members, advocacy organizations, and other nonclinical support services (i.e., housing and peer support services) that interface with the behavioral health system.

Family beliefs about tobacco use influence whether individuals with behavioral health conditions try to quit and access treatment. As with other groups, having family or peers with negative views about tobacco and nonsmoking family and friends is associated with more quitting behaviors, including the use of tobacco treatment medications (Nagawa et al. 2022). Interventions to educate family and integrate them into the tobacco treatment plan could provide additional support and enhance success. Complicating this is that family caregivers of people with behavioral health conditions may still perceive the distribution of tobacco as part of their caring role (Lawn et al. 2015). Similarly, advocacy organizations in the past were ambivalent about addressing tobacco and too often relied on misinformation and "myths" that tobacco was a reasonable reward or coping strategy (Solway 2011).

Individuals with mental illness are likely to live with other tobacco users and continue to smoke indoors (Metse et al. 2016). Since 2016, the U.S. Department of Housing and Urban Development has mandated that public housing developments in the United States be smoke-free because secondhand smoke in multi-unit dwellings cannot be contained and adversely effects the health of everyone in that space. Although a full review of tobacco-free housing is beyond the scope of this book, it remains an important target for strengthening and supporting efforts for helping individuals with behavioral health conditions to quit smoking. Staff in residential and housing programs can strengthen the efforts of the health care team and provide support for tobacco-free activities and alternatives.

There are many ways that peer counselors can influence tobacco use and help to change norms around using tobacco in the behavioral health community. The peer support model is based on shared responsibility, respect, and mutual understanding of what is helpful, and peers are able to discuss tobacco in a less threatening way to those fearful of change. Seeing peers who are in tobacco recovery provides role models and hope to others. In this way, peers may have greater success in reaching people who are not motivated to discuss changing their tobacco use. Advantages of using peer counselors include reduced language and cultural barriers, increased trust and lowered defenses, and lower cost.

Successful peer models for addressing tobacco use have been described (Williams et al. 2011; see also njchoices.org); some employ former tobacco users with lived experience of mental illness who are provided training in TUD and community outreach. In addition to providing education and a message of hope, peer counselors can often lead mutual self-help groups to provide additional support and supplement the treatment effort and to provide a brief assessment and intervention that includes referral to another service, such as a telephone quitline (Baker et al. 2019).

Case Example

A large substance abuse program that has a range of outpatient and residential services is thinking of establishing tobacco-free grounds on the property. The staff have organized to express their grievances because they are concerned that this will negatively impact them as well as the patients. Currently, the facility has no restrictions on tobacco use, and staff often smoke alongside patients during breaks. They believe it will be disruptive to patients to make them abstain from tobacco during other SUD treatment.

What Are the Concerns in This Case?

This is a common scenario, and many of the staff concerns have been refuted in research studies. Staff should be given access to education, reassurance, and support as the organization undergoes changes. Staff using tobacco should be treated with compassion and given access to resources and additional support. Tobacco causes many consequences for individuals with SUD, including leading to more deaths than even their primary drug. Continued tobacco use is also associated with more relapse back to drug and alcohol use. Patients in SUD treatment are receptive to treatment for tobacco use and recognize it as an addiction.

Tobacco-free grounds in behavioral health treatment programs have not resulted in patients not coming to or signing out of treatment. Even when patients are not willing to make a long-term commitment to abstinence from tobacco, it can still be a worthwhile experience for them to undergo a safe and comfortable detoxification from tobacco while receiving other SUD treatment. This period of temporary abstinence is consistent with program goals to practice a lifestyle that does not rely on drugs, including tobacco, for coping. All patients in these settings should have access to medications that reduce the experience of tobacco withdrawal symptoms. A positive experience can help people be more willing to try tobacco treatment in the future. The program can emphasize the positive aspects of how systems changes enhance care for deadly tobacco addiction and reduce cues and triggers in the environment. At the very least, efforts should be taken to restrict staff and patients smoking together because practicing this addiction should not be a shared activity.

Key Points

- Implementing systems changes in the clinical environment is an evidence-based practice that increases access to treatments for tobacco use disorder and supplements these clinical practices.
- All staff can participate in brief interventions such as screening, but having designated staff with additional training and expertise can be helpful to provide evidence-based clinical treatments.
- Tobacco use can be integrated into other work in behavioral health treatment settings using the co-occurring disorders model, which supports that every interaction is an opportunity to talk about tobacco use and that interventions should not be reserved for only those wanting to quit.
- Policies that restrict tobacco use completely in the environment (i.e., tobacco-free treatment grounds) are effective. Even in the absence of this type of policy change, other policies can be developed that support treatment and health behaviors.
- Assisting staff who use tobacco to access support and treatment sends a consistent and compassionate message that addressing tobacco is essential for everyone.

References

Baker AL, Borland R, Bonevski B, et al: "Quitlink": a randomized controlled trial of peer worker facilitated quitline support for smokers receiving mental health services: study protocol. Front Psychiatry 10:124, 2019 30941063

Bernstein SM, Stoduto G: Adding a choice-based program for tobacco smoking to an abstinence-based addiction treatment program. J Subst Abuse Treat 17(1–2):167–173, 1999

Braun BL, Fowles JB, Solberg LI, et al: Smoking-related attitudes and clinical practices of medical personnel in Minnesota. Am J Prev Med 27(4):316–322, 2004

Brown E, Nonnemaker J, Federman EB, et al: Implementation of a tobacco-free regulation in substance use disorder treatment facilities. J Subst Abuse Treat 42(3):319–327, 2012 22000325

Brown RA, Minami H, Hecht J, et al: Sustained care smoking cessation intervention for individuals hospitalized for psychiatric disorders: the Helping Hand 3 randomized clinical trial. JAMA Psychiatry 78(8):839–847, 2021

Buchanan C, Nahhas GJ, Guille C, et al: Tobacco use prevalence and outcomes among perinatal patients assessed through an "opt-out" cessation and follow-up clinical program. Matern Child Health J 21(9):1790–1797, 2017 28702864

Burke MV, Ebbert JO, Schroeder DR, et al: Treatment outcomes from a specialist model for treating tobacco use disorder in a medical center. Medicine (Baltimore) 94(44):e1903, 2015 26554789

Burns A, Gutta J, Kooreman H, et al: Strategic use of tobacco treatment specialists as an innovation for tobacco cessation health systems change within health care organizations. Health Care Manage Rev 48(4):323–333, 2023 37615942

Campbell BK, Le T, McCuistian C, et al: Implementing tobacco-free policy in residential substance use disorders treatment: practice changes among staff. Drug Alcohol Depend Rep 2:100033, 2022 36845887

Carson KV, Verbiest MEA, Crone MR, et al: Training health professionals in smoking cessation. Cochrane Database Syst Rev 2012(5):CD000214, 2012 22592671

Centers for Disease Control and Prevention: Best Practices for Comprehensive Tobacco Control Programs. Washington, DC, U.S. Department of Health and Human Services, 2014. Available at: https://www.cdc.gov/tobacco/stateandcommunity/guides/pdfs/2014/comprehensive.pdf. Accessed August 5, 2024.

Covell NH, Foster F, Lipton N, et al: Self-evaluation tool to support implementation of treatment for tobacco use disorder in behavioral health programs. Community Ment Health J 58(4):812–820, 2022 34518927

Friedmann PD, Jiang L, Richter KP: Cigarette smoking cessation services in outpatient substance abuse treatment programs in the United States. J Subst Abuse Treat 34(2):165–172, 2008 17509809

Guydish J, Le T, Hosakote S, et al: Tobacco use among substance use disorder (SUD) treatment staff is associated with tobacco-related services received by clients. J Subst Abuse Treat 132:108496, 2022 34111773

Hahn EJ, Warnick TA, Plemmons S: Smoking cessation in drug treatment programs. J Addict Dis 18(4):89–101, 1999

Hehir AM, Indig D, Prosser S, et al: Implementation of a smoke-free policy in a high secure mental health inpatient facility: staff survey to describe experience and attitudes. BMC Public Health 13:315, 2013 23566256

Hoffman AL, Slade J: Following the pioneers: addressing tobacco in chemical dependency treatment. J Subst Abuse Treat 10(2):153–160, 1993 8389896

Lawn S, Campion J: Achieving smoke-free mental health services: lessons from the past decade of implementation research. Int J Environ Res Public Health 10(9):4224–4244, 2013 24025397

Lawn S, Pols R: Smoking bans in psychiatric inpatient settings? A review of the research. Aust N Z J Psychiatry 39(10):866–885, 2005 16168014

Lawn S, McNaughton D, Fuller L: What carers of family members with mental illness say, think and do about their relative's smoking and the implications for health promotion and service delivery: a qualitative study. Int J Ment Health Promot 17(5):261–277, 2015

Marynak K, VanFrank B, Tetlow S, et al: Tobacco cessation interventions and smoke-free policies in mental health and substance abuse treatment facilities—United States, 2016. MMWR Morb Mortal Wkly Rep 67(18):519–523, 2018 29746451

McEwen A, West R, McRobbie H: Effectiveness of specialist group treatment for smoking cessation vs. one-to-one treatment in primary care. Addict Behav 31(9):1650–1660, 2006 16443331

Meredith LS, Yano EM, Hickey SC, et al: Primary care provider attitudes are associated with smoking cessation counseling and referral. Med Care 43(9):929–934, 2005 16116358

Metse AP, Wiggers J, Wye P, et al: Smoking and environmental characteristics of smokers with a mental illness, and associations with quitting behaviour and motivation; a cross sectional study. BMC Public Health 16:332, 2016 27080019

Metse AP, Wiggers J, Wye P, et al: Efficacy of a universal smoking cessation intervention initiated in inpatient psychiatry and continued post-discharge: a randomised controlled trial. Aust N Z J Psychiatry 51(4):366–381, 2017 28195010

Nagawa CS, Wang B, Davis M, et al: Examining pathways between family or peer factors and smoking cessation in a nationally representative US sample of adults with mental health conditions who smoke: a structural equation analysis. BMC Public Health 22(1):1566, 2022 35978318

Nahhas GJ, Wilson D, Talbot V, et al: Feasibility of implementing a hospital-based "opt-out" tobacco-cessation service. Nicotine Tob Res 19(8):937–943, 2017 27928052

Prochaska JJ, Hall SE, Delucchi K, et al: Efficacy of initiating tobacco dependence treatment in inpatient psychiatry: a randomized controlled trial. Am J Public Health 104(8):1557–1565, 2014 23948001

Ratschen E, Britton J, Doody GA, et al: Tobacco dependence, treatment and smoke-free policies: a survey of mental health professionals' knowledge and attitudes. Gen Hosp Psychiatry 31(6):576–582, 2009 19892217

Riad-Allen L, Dermody SS, Herman Y, et al: Becoming tobacco-free: changes in staff and patient attitudes and incident reports in a large academic mental health and addictions hospital. Am J Addict 26(2):183–191, 2017 28211960

Richter KP, Ellerbeck EF: It's time to change the default for tobacco treatment. Addiction 110(3):381–386, 2015 25323093

Richter KP, Hunt JJ, Cupertino AP, et al: Understanding the drug treatment community's ambivalence towards tobacco use and treatment. Int J Drug Policy 23(3):220–228, 2012 22280918

Scheeres A, Xhezo R, Julius R, et al: Changes in voluntary admission and restraint use after a comprehensive tobacco-free policy in inpatient psychiatric health facilities. Subst Abus 41(2):252–258, 2020 31295085

Sheffer CE, Al-Zalabani A, Aubrey A, et al: The emerging global tobacco treatment workforce: characteristics of tobacco treatment specialists trained in council-accredited training programs from 2017 to 2019. Int J Environ Res Public Health 18(5):2416, 2021 33801227

Shi Y, Cummins SE: Smoking cessation services and smoke-free policies at substance abuse treatment facilities: national survey results. Psychiatr Serv 66(6):610–616, 2015 25686819

Shoesmith E, Huddlestone L, Lorencatto F, et al: Supporting smoking cessation and preventing relapse following a stay in a smoke-free setting: a meta-analysis and investigation of effective behaviour change techniques. Addiction 116(11):2978–2994, 2021 33620737

Slater P, McElwee G, Fleming P, et al: Nurses' smoking behaviour related to cessation practice. Nurs Times 102(19):32–37, 2006

Solway ES: The lived experiences of tobacco use, dependence, and cessation: insights and perspectives of people with mental illness. Health Soc Work 36(1):19–32, 2011 21446606

Substance Abuse and Mental Health Services Administration: Tobacco cessation services. The N-SSATS Report, September 19, 2013. Available at: https://www.samhsa.gov/data/sites/default/files/N-SSATS%20Rprt%20Tobacco%20Cessation%20Services/The%20N-SSATS%20Report%20%20Tobacco%20Cessation%20Services/The%20N-SSATS%20Report%20%20Tobacco%20Cessation%20Services.htm. Accessed August 5, 2024.

Substance Abuse and Mental Health Services Administration: 2020 National Mental Health Services Survey (N-MHSS) Annual Report. Rockville, MD, Substance Abuse and Mental Health Services Administration, 2020. Available at: https://www.samhsa.gov/data/report/national-mental -health-services-survey-n-mhss-2020-data-mental-health-treatment -facilities. Accessed August 5, 2024.

Tong EK, Strouse R, Hall J, et al: National survey of U.S. health professionals' smoking prevalence, cessation practices, and beliefs. Nicotine Tob Res 12(7):724–733, 2010 20507899

U.S. Department of Health and Human Services: Smoking Cessation: A Report of the Surgeon General. Atlanta, GA, U.S. Department of Health and Human Services, Centers for Disease Control and Prevention, National Center for Chronic Disease Prevention and Health Promotion, Office on Smoking and Health, 2020

Voci S, Bondy S, Zawertailo L, et al: Impact of a smoke-free policy in a large psychiatric hospital on staff attitudes and patient behavior. Gen Hosp Psychiatry 32(6):623–630, 2010 21112455

Williams JM: Eliminating tobacco use in mental health facilities: patients' rights, public health, and policy issues. JAMA 299(5):571–573, 2008 18252888

Williams JM, Foulds J, Dwyer M, et al: The integration of tobacco dependence treatment and tobacco-free standards into residential addictions treatment in New Jersey. J Subst Abuse Treat 28(4):331–340, 2005 15925267

Williams JM, Dwyer M, Verna M, et al: Evaluation of the CHOICES program of peer-to-peer tobacco education and advocacy. Community Ment Health J 47(3):243–251, 2011 20419349

Williams JM, Miskimen T, Minsky S, et al: Increasing tobacco dependence treatment through continuing education training for behavioral health professionals. Psychiatr Serv 66(1):21–26, 2015 25220158

Williams JM, Poulsen R, Chaguturu V, et al: Evaluation of an online residency training in tobacco use disorder. Am J Addict 28(4):277–284, 2019 30993797

Young WJ, Delnevo CD, Singh B, et al: Tobacco treatment knowledge and practices among US psychiatrists. Community Ment Health J 59(1):185–191, 2023 35768703

11

Addressing Mental Illness and Other Substance Use During Treatment for Tobacco Use Disorder

There are some unique issues to consider when helping individuals with behavioral health comorbidity address their tobacco use. As has been discussed in previous chapters, this population experiences many challenges yet is largely motivated to quit, and the changing culture and attitudes from providers and treatment centers toward addressing tobacco use are likely contributing to recent reductions in overall smoking rates among these groups. Despite these modest advances, however, large disparities continue to exist, and more people with behavioral health conditions who also smoke need to receive evidence-based treatments to help them quit. Given the patterns of heavy smoking, higher severity of tobacco use disorder (TUD), normalization of using tobacco to cope, and lower quit rates in this population, special considerations can be made and approaches to treatment can be taken that may enhance abstinence outcomes. Although discussed here, these sorts of modifications are modest, and these groups, like any other tobacco users, are more likely to benefit from receiving the previously described evidence-based treatments.

Some of the specific clinical issues of subpopulations (e.g., people with anxiety disorders or schizophrenia) are also discussed here, with an emphasis on the implications for treatment. A complicating factor in understanding the literature is distinctions between tobacco users with current versus past or lifetime mental disorders. Current or persistent illness likely presents additional challenges and is more common in the clinical setting. Illness severity and functional impairment may ultimately be more important prognostic factors than discrete diagnostic subgroups because there is considerable overlap in diagnoses. It is also common for individuals to have more than one type of behavioral health condition, limiting the generalizability of some studies (using single diagnoses) and making analyses of mixed diagnostic groups (i.e., those with serious psychological distress [SPD]) that measure recent impairment and distress important to consider as well. Recent studies show a rise in SPD in the United States, and adults with substance use disorder (SUD) who smoke cigarettes are twice as likely to also have SPD as those who do not smoke cigarettes (Parker et al. 2021). This shows that comorbidity of mental illness and SUD is the norm, not the exception, and treatments ideally should address the intersectionality of all three (tobacco, mental illness, and SUD).

Overall Impact on Cessation

Many studies have shown reduced success in quitting smoking among patients with some type of behavioral health condition. This includes data from clinical trials as well as epidemiological samples that looked at quit ratios, or quitting behavior, over time. Perhaps the best data come from the large Evaluating Adverse Events in a Global Smoking Cessation Study (EAGLES), which demonstrated that people with any current and/or lifetime mood, anxiety, or psychotic illness who also smoke achieved lower 3-month and 6-month abstinence rates compared with people without such diagnoses who smoke (Anthenelli et al. 2016; West et al. 2018). Strengths of this study include the large sample size and use of structured diagnostic interviews to confirm the presence or absence of mental illness (EAGLES is discussed in more detail in Chapter 7). Studies of people with serious mental illness (SMI), which typically refers to those with bipolar disorder, schizophrenia, or severe major depression, consistently show reduced smoking cessation on a given quit attempt and lower lifetime quit ratios (Fornaro et al. 2022; Glasheen et al. 2014). The data for milder anxiety and mood disorders are more mixed and sometimes do not distinguish between past/lifetime or current illness. Conditions that are generally more severe or involve persistent symptoms, such as PTSD, can be associated with reduced quit rates compared with episodic illnesses such as panic disorder (PD). Illness severity is likely the mitigating factor associated with greater tobacco use severity and subsequently more difficulty quitting across all of these conditions.

Treatments have been widely studied in people with SUD, including those with alcohol or drug dependence. A meta-analysis of trials indicates efficacy for medications as well as combinations of medications and counseling in SUD populations (Apollonio et al. 2016). Counseling-only approaches did not significantly increase tobacco abstinence and, like trials in SMI populations, support the idea that this is a heavily tobacco-dependent group that needs medication to be successful in quitting. Tobacco treatments are effective for people in early treatment as well as those in longer recovery with sustained abstinence from other substances (Joseph et al. 2004).

Impact on Symptoms

Many studies have demonstrated that trying to quit smoking does not worsen, and may even improve, symptoms of mental illness (Taylor et al. 2021). This implies that there is no wrong time to try to quit tobacco if the person is ready to do so, as long as there are no safety concerns that would interfere, such as dangerous or severely disorganized thoughts or behavior. Patients often believe that the clinical symptoms of tobacco withdrawal, which can include restlessness, anxiety, and trouble sleeping, are evidence of their recurring mental illness. However, if they receive adequate pharmacological treatment for tobacco withdrawal, these symptoms should be lessened, and the patient can be reassured. Tobacco withdrawal symptoms that can mimic symptoms of another anxiety or mood disorder often improve within 6 weeks of abstinence, and studies show that patients report reduced symptoms of depression and anxiety after quitting, compared with baseline (Taylor et al. 2014). Tobacco withdrawal symptoms can emerge within hours of the last cigarette, are worse in the morning, and occur intermittently throughout the day, even on typical smoking days. This implies that even some of the day-to-day fluctuating symptoms that patients experience might be caused by the short-lived effects of nicotine peaks and troughs associated with smoking and withdrawal. Even brief periods of tobacco withdrawal (a few hours), then, could be clinically significant and cause the person distress and feelings of anger, irritability, or anxiety.

Although early case reports suggested varenicline caused agitation, depression, and suicidal ideation, these findings were not borne out in many large placebo-controlled trials and database analyses. In the EAGLES, people with psychiatric illness who also smoked were more likely to report moderate to severe neuropsychiatric adverse events, although these were not related to the medication they received (Anthenelli et al. 2019). This may have occurred for two reasons. First, this group often has higher measures of smoking heaviness and TUD severity, which implies more frequent and severe tobacco withdrawal symptoms that could be misattributed to medication side effects. Second, reports of these side effects may be related to underlying mental illness, stress, or some other reason.

Importantly, studies of patients with psychotic illnesses such as schizophrenia show no worsening of psychotic symptoms during an attempt to quit smoking, regardless of whether the person is successful in quitting (Tsoi et al. 2013; Williams et al. 2012). One study of people with schizophrenia who smoked showed a clinically significant reduction in agitation associated with the use of the 21-mg nicotine patch when patients were treated in an emergency department setting (Allen et al. 2011), again underscoring that tobacco withdrawal symptoms can mimic other disorders and should always be treated during periods of (even brief) temporary abstinence.

Impact on Quitting and Modifications to Treatment

Many, but not all, behavioral health conditions have been associated with greater difficulty quitting smoking and less success in a given attempt. A variety of biopsychosocial factors may contribute to this (discussed in Chapter 5). Biological factors include higher measures of smoking heaviness and TUD severity and more frequent and severe tobacco withdrawal symptoms. Psychological factors include many components, such as attitudes and beliefs about tobacco or quitting, motivation and readiness to change, and ability to cope with distress. Social factors can also undermine quitting success if someone lives with someone or has many friends who use tobacco or does not have a tobacco-free living space. A thorough assessment that includes a relapse analysis of past attempts can help identify issues that may have undermined those attempts. Being aware of common cues and triggers and helping the patient avoid or cope with these can enhance success. Counseling and medication treatments address many of these barriers but also can be tailored to the unique needs of the individual.

In terms of medications, a few adaptations might be made for those with behavioral health comorbidity, although, in general, other best practices (i.e., varenicline or combination nicotine replacement therapy [NRT] as first-line treatment) still apply. The EAGLES tested varenicline, bupropion, and nicotine patch monotherapy versus placebo in more than 4,000 people who smoked and who also had confirmed mental illness. Abstinence rates with varenicline were superior to the other medication groups among the subgroups with psychotic, mood, and anxiety disorders (Evins et al. 2019), supporting its role as a first-line treatment. Combination NRT similarly is a good choice given its superiority to NRT monotherapy in clinical trials and makes good clinical sense given the heavier tobacco use and higher levels of dependence in these patient groups. Nicotine medication, which has none of the toxins associated with tobacco and smoking, can be thought of as a low-risk intervention that could be useful for almost every tobacco user, even in situations where aftercare may be compromised and follow-up uncertain. This is supported by its over-the-counter (OTC) classification. Because nicotine and varenicline have no clinically significant medication interactions in the liver, they can be safely given with other psychiatric medications. Bupropion can also be safe in these populations, although it is contraindicated in people with a seizure disorder or active eating disorder and has the potential to interact with medications metabolized by the hepatic enzymes CYP2B6 and CYP2D6.

Counseling modifications for behavioral health populations include more sessions, more motivational counseling, and greater flexibility in setting the quit date. Both individual and group treatment can be effective. Counseling alone is less likely to be successful and should always be combined with pharmacotherapy. Telephone quitlines are developing protocols that include these modifications for callers with behavioral health comorbidity. Other helpful approaches could include encouraging participation in peer-led support groups or providing additional contacts through supplementary phone calls. Tobacco dependence can be viewed as a chronic condition requiring a long-term treatment approach, and relapse is common. Even in the general population, few people are successful in their first quit attempt, and most require numerous attempts before they succeed. In a specialty tobacco treatment clinic, patients who returned for repeat treatment were more likely to have a history of mental illness (Han et al. 2006). Working with patients for a period of 2–3 years to achieve sustained abstinence is not uncommon (Williams and Foulds 2007). These repeated attempts, often with weeks of abstinence, can reduce overall exposure to tobacco toxins and lead to eventual successful quitting. Behavioral health practitioners take a long-term approach to treating other co-occurring mental health and addictions disorders, a model that also may be useful for treating tobacco use. Integrating tobacco dependence treatment into other treatments for behavioral health conditions may be more effective than other strategies and makes the most sense (McFall et al. 2010).

Timing of Treatment

The timing of tobacco use treatment is something that is still debated in some behavioral health settings. It can be advantageous to address tobacco use during early SUD treatment, especially in a protected treatment setting such as an inpatient or residential detoxification or treatment program. Addressing all substances, including tobacco, is consistent with the overall treatment philosophy of a drug-free lifestyle. A structured environment that is focused on recovery allows for ample staff and peer support as well as access to medications to address withdrawal. Many studies have shown that patients are interested in addressing tobacco use while receiving other SUD treatment (Prochaska et al. 2004a; Richter et al. 2002). Drug craving and exposure to smoking cues can trigger the use of other substances and undermine recovery and other abstinence goals. Success rates for quitting smoking during early substance recovery are comparable with those achieved when treatment is delayed for 6 months (Joseph et al. 2004), and most studies show that providing concurrent smoking cessation treatment does not worsen and can even improve outcomes for the primary substance (Apollonio et al. 2016; McKelvey et al. 2017; Thurgood et al. 2016; Winhusen et al. 2014). Intervening during a psychiatric hospitalization with a brief approach consisting of motivational counseling, free patches at discharge, and free telephone/text follow-up resulted in almost three times as many people quitting at 6 months (Brown et al. 2021).

In tobacco-free settings such as inpatient or residential treatment centers, it is reasonable to frame the treatment as temporary abstinence and an opportunity for safe and comfortable detoxification from all substances, including tobacco. Patients need not commit to abstinence after discharge to benefit from learning about the consequences of tobacco use and the benefits of treatment. In the same way, tobacco use can also be addressed during a psychiatric inpatient hospitalization. This can even provide an opportunity for a supported detox from tobacco that would not be possible otherwise. Inpatient studies have shown that early discharges are reduced and lengths of stay are longer when patients are given access to adequate nicotine replacement while in the hospital (Prochaska et al. 2004b), which underscores the clinical significance of tobacco withdrawal and the need for treatment in all settings. An emergency department study had similar findings; patients with schizophrenia who received a 21-mg nicotine patch in the emergency department were significantly less agitated than those who had received a placebo. The reduction in agitation was clinically significant and comparable with the effect seen from a dose of antipsychotic medication (Allen et al. 2011).

Impact on Behavioral Health Conditions

Depression

Both clinical and epidemiological studies show that individuals with depression smoke at higher rates, are more dependent, and have more difficulty quitting and higher relapse rates (Weinberger et al. 2017b). Although they do not have differences in their motivation to quit compared with people without depression (Siru et al. 2009), they do report smoking more to relieve negative affect and experiencing more symptoms of withdrawal during a quit attempt (Weinberger et al. 2010). Different beliefs endorsed by people with depression can have important impacts on quitting behavior and treatment outcomes. Smoking interventions that address mood and include mood management strategies yield better outcomes than standard interventions in people with depression (van der Meer et al. 2013). Mood management adaptations include cognitive-behavioral therapy (CBT) techniques focused on behavioral activation, cognitive restructuring, and social skills training and can be adapted for telephone counseling sessions. These CBT-based strategies help patients manage the affective distress associated with quitting smoking by improving coping skills, increasing positive activities, and minimizing relapse-related negative thoughts (Haas et al. 2004).

Two antidepressants, bupropion and nortriptyline, have been shown to be effective for quitting smoking, although nortriptyline use is often limited by side effects, including weight gain. Although they are effective even in people without depression, they can be a preferred option for people with depression who want one medication treatment that addresses both mood and tobacco use. However, evidence from recent studies indicates that varenicline is superior to bupropion for tobacco use treatment, even in people with depression (Howes et al. 2020).

Schizophrenia, Bipolar Disorder, and Other Serious Mental Illnesses

People with schizophrenia tend to smoke more and have greater dependence than other people who smoke. The strong association between schizophrenia and higher rates of smoking has been shown worldwide (de Leon and Diaz 2005). There is also evidence of more intense smoking patterns in this group, as well as more use of a rapid, shallow puffing pattern that is linked to higher nicotine intake per cigarette (Williams et al. 2011). The "self-medication" hypothesis in schizophrenia suggests that higher nicotine intake is needed to compensate for the abnormal nicotinic cholinergic systems that are linked to attention and cognition through sensory gating and reward learning. An alternate view is that abnormal dopaminergic and other neurotransmitter systems in schizophrenia are linked with a heightened risk of all SUDs (Berg et al. 2014; Chambers 2013), which is consistent with studies showing high intake of other substances, including caffeine (Rosen et al. 2023). Recent studies have also provided strong evidence that smoking in patients with schizophrenia is linked with worse (not better) cognitive functioning and more impairment compared with schizophrenic patients who never smoked or previously smoked (Coustals et al. 2020; Mallet et al. 2022).

All of the FDA-approved medications for tobacco use have been shown to be effective in people with schizophrenia or other psychotic disorders. Interestingly, the quit rates in the placebo groups of these studies often show very low abstinence rates, supporting the idea that behavioral support alone is inadequate and that these patients need medication to be successful. In laboratory studies, people with schizophrenia who also smoked reported more severe cigarette craving and nicotine withdrawal symptoms during a 72-hour abstinence period and greater relapse to smoking compared with control subjects matched for level of dependence (Tidey et al. 2014). Counseling approaches often are modified to address the cognitive issues related to schizophrenia; modifications may include more sessions, flexible quit dates, and a slower, more supportive pace, as well as more education, such as written handouts, to reinforce key concepts (Williams et al. 2010). Both group and individual counseling approaches can be helpful. Monetary incentives provided as reward for biological confirmation of abstinence (exhaled carbon monoxide level) can also be effective when combined with treatment (Brunette et al. 2018).

Fewer studies of people with bipolar disorder are available, but smoking among these individuals has been associated with more severe (mood and psychotic) symptoms, other SUDs, and suicide attempts (Corvin et al. 2001; Heffner et al. 2011; Vanable et al. 2003). Smoking cessation is achievable, although these factors present challenges and can make quitting more difficult. Patients can benefit similarly from pharmacotherapy. The risk for mania from bupropion is a consideration, but this risk is thought to be lower with bupropion than with other antidepressants (Pacchiarotti et al. 2013). Anecdotal information suggests that tobacco use behavior may vary with symptom cycling, increasing with episodes of severe depression or mania, and longitudinal studies are needed to help determine the best time for bipolar disorder patients to attempt quitting. The efficacy of varenicline in this population was higher than that for bupropion or nicotine patch (Heffner et al. 2019).

Longer durations of tobacco use treatment also may be needed in people with schizophrenia or bipolar disorder. One study showed a high risk for relapse back to smoking for participants whose varenicline was stopped after 3 months compared with a group that received it for a full year (Evins et al. 2014). Interestingly, even at the end of the year when the medication was withdrawn, relapse to smoking seemed rapid, suggesting that even longer, maintenance-type medications may be needed. Longer durations of medications for TUD are safe and well tolerated, and this maintenance approach is consistent with other medications for addictions treatment, which often may be given for years.

Given the clinical overlap between psychiatric diagnoses, some studies have included groups of people across a spectrum of SMI, which implies significant functional impairment and, often, a chronic component to the mental illness symptoms. SPD based on the K6 (Kessler et al. 2002; discussed in Chapter 5) provides a good estimate of SMI in population studies. Medications are warranted for different SMI disorder subtypes. Smoking interventions for people with SMI include adaptations to psychosocial counseling to address cognitive and motivational issues, as described earlier (Gilbody et al. 2019). Learning About Healthy Living (LAHL) is a treatment approach that was developed for working with seriously mentally ill patients who may not be immediately ready to commit to tobacco abstinence (Williams et al. 2009). Discussed in Chapter 8, LAHL is an easy-to-implement group treatment that frames tobacco within an overall approach to healthy living that educates tobacco users about the consequences of use and options for treatment without requiring a commitment to abstinence. It can be conceptualized as a pre-cessation curriculum that can help increase the demand for tobacco treatment services and is available in the public domain (https://rwjms.rutgers.edu/sites/default/files/2024-04/2012_lahl.pdf).

Individuals with SMI are also less successful in quitting using telephone counseling services, often called quitlines. Modifications to the usual quitline format may enhance outcomes in this group, such as using the same counselor for every call from a given patient, linking with the behavioral health treatment team, and increasing the number of calls or time to discuss NRT (Baker et al. 2019; Carpenter et al. 2019). Having peers facilitate referrals and call patients proactively may also be helpful ways to enhance quitline use.

Anxiety Disorders

Similar to people with other mental illnesses, individuals with anxiety disorders smoke at higher rates and in higher amounts and have more tobacco use severity (Garey et al. 2020). They have earlier and more severe withdrawal symptoms when attempting to quit (Piper et al. 2011) and reduced success in quitting. They also report stress and negative affect as precursors to relapse and seem to have greater fear around the somatic experience of quitting.

In one study, individuals with anxiety disorders (PD, generalized anxiety disorder [GAD], or PTSD) were more likely than those without psychiatric illness to experience moderate to severe neuropsychiatric adverse effects during a smoking cessation attempt regardless of medication treatment group (varenicline vs. bupropion vs. patch vs. placebo) (Ayers et al. 2020). People with PTSD reported the most adverse events, and reports of sleep disturbance, anxiety, and gastrointestinal events were common across all anxiety disorder subgroups. Another study showed a lack of nicotine or bupropion medication efficacy (compared with placebo) in people with anxiety disorders (panic attacks, social anxiety, or GAD), although this has not been replicated (Piper et al. 2011). Experiencing more than one anxiety disorder, PTSD, or comorbid depression is also associated with reduced tobacco abstinence.

Although they are often grouped together, these diagnostic subgroups may have important differences that affect their response to tobacco treatments. PD and PTSD may have a larger somatic component (vs. cognitive worrying, as in GAD) that complicates the experience of withdrawal and quitting. Data from the EAGLES showed that varenicline was effective for smoking cessation in participants with GAD and PD, whereas NRT provided significant benefit for those with PD (Ayers et al. 2020). Although data are limited, they suggest that bupropion could be ineffective and may produce more side effects in people with PD or PTSD; this is consistent with other data in PD indicating that these individuals have higher pre-quit levels of craving, negative affect, and anxiety around the anticipation of quitting that easily can be confused with tobacco withdrawal symptoms and thus perhaps more responsive to NRT. Anxiolytics have not been found to be helpful for quitting tobacco (Hughes et al. 2000).

Impact on Other Substance Use and Substance Use Disorder

Tobacco use overlaps with and influences substance use and SUD in a variety of biopsychosocial ways. Common brain pathways are activated by nicotine and other drugs, and nicotine's ability to enhance reward in the brain is similar to that of other drugs. Behaviors and cues can be similar or overlapping, especially if other drugs are also smoked. Smoking relapse risk is increased among individuals in recovery from other substance use (Quisenberry et al. 2019). Treatment consensus is that abstinence from all substances, versus only some, produces the best outcomes and reduces the risk for relapse. This can be challenging because motivational levels may differ regarding different substances. Co-users of tobacco and cannabis, for example, are often more motivated to stop using tobacco than cannabis (McClure et al. 2019). Specific information about individual substances is discussed in the sections that follow.

Alcohol

Even recent studies show that cigarette use remains twice as common among people with alcohol use disorder (AUD) than among those without AUD (Weinberger et al. 2019), with no difference due to AUD severity. Quit rates for those with past-year AUD are about half those seen in people without AUD (Weinberger et al. 2017a). Similar trends are seen among individuals who are heavy alcohol users but who may not meet the criteria for AUD and translate into less quitting over these patients' lifetimes. Concurrent alcohol use also seems to undermine tobacco quit attempts in a dose-dependent way (van Amsterdam and van den Brink 2023).

There are limited studies examining quit attempts and specific components of quitting behavior in AUD populations. The largest study was a clinical trial of 499 people with AUD that compared concurrent (during intensive alcohol treatment) or delayed (6 months later) tobacco use treatment (Joseph et al. 2004). Participants in the concurrent group were more likely to participate in treatment, although quit rates did not differ between the groups at 18-month follow-up. Alcohol abstinence was slightly worse in the concurrent group, although this study has not been replicated, and a recent meta-analysis of 34 studies showed no worsening of SUD outcomes with tobacco treatment (Apollonio et al. 2016). An important consideration is that individuals with AUD are more likely to die from tobacco effects (Hurt et al. 1996), and delayed treatment may not be available in a real (non-research) setting. The risks of continued smoking and the lower quit rates seen in epidemiological studies support the need for integrated tobacco treatment during other SUD treatment. Clinical studies have shown that people who smoke who have been in alcohol recovery for 1 year or more are just as likely to quit as other people who smoke (Hughes and Callas 2003), which is notable because they may smoke more and have higher levels of dependence. However, they have experience quitting substances, which may be an advantage that helps them quit successfully despite their higher levels of dependence.

Studies have shown that nicotine replacement or varenicline can be effective (Apollonio et al. 2016; Guo et al. 2021). Varenicline may offer advantages in AUD populations because it modifies dopamine reward pathways and reduces the rewarding effects of alcohol. Excreted in the urine, it also does not affect the liver or liver enzymes. Patients who smoke who are treated with varenicline experience an anti-craving effect and significantly reduce alcohol consumption (Oon-Arom et al. 2019). Varenicline's effects on reducing alcohol use seem greatest among people who smoke and are heavy drinkers, compared with people who do not smoke (Fischler et al. 2022; Mitchell et al. 2012). Naltrexone is not effective for tobacco cessation.

Cannabis

Co-use of cannabis and tobacco is of increasing importance because daily cannabis use has increased overwhelmingly in recent years among people who also smoke cigarettes (Goodwin et al. 2018). Cannabis users have higher tobacco smoking rates (Weinberger et al. 2021), which is further complicated by the use of mixed tobacco and cannabis products, such as spliffs (tobacco rolled with marijuana), blunts (cannabis wrapped in a tobacco leaf), or vaporizers. Smoking still produces products of combustion, such as carbon monoxide, making it more difficult to verify abstinence using patients' exhaled carbon monoxide measurements.

Use of both cannabis and tobacco can impact individuals negatively in several ways, such as contributing to worse mental and physical health, a higher risk for SUDs, and more difficulty quitting (Fitzke et al. 2022). Motivational levels may differ for the substances used, and users often increase drug substitution, using more of one when trying to quit the other (McClure et al. 2019). Clinically, there is considerable overlap in withdrawal symptoms from these substances, with both causing irritability, anxiety, depressed mood, insomnia, and restlessness (American Psychiatric Association 2022; see Table 11–1). To date, few trials have studied use of both cannabis and tobacco, and many questions persist about how sex and mental health comorbidity may impact outcomes.

Although patients may not be motivated to address cannabis use while working on quitting tobacco, it can still undermine their success in the tobacco quit attempt. Quit ratios, which measure likelihood of becoming a "former smoker," are lower for cannabis users (23% vs. 51% for no cannabis use) and lower still for those with cannabis use disorder (Weinberger et al. 2020). Daily cannabis users are less likely to quit smoking using a telephone tobacco quitline (Goodwin et al. 2022). A study of varenicline for smoking cessation in young people (ages 14–21 years) found that 59% had a positive urine drug screen for cannabinoids at baseline (Gray et al. 2019), and cannabis users in this trial were half as likely to quit smoking (McClure et al. 2020). Similarly, trials of medications for cannabis use disorder show reduced success in patients who smoke tobacco (Gray et al. 2017). Few trials have looked at the simultaneous quitting of tobacco and cannabis and the acceptability of this to patients, although it makes clinical sense.

Opioids and Other Drug Use Disorders

Tobacco use rates among opioid users are among the highest reported for any diagnostic subgroup, and this leads to high rates of morbidity and premature death. Quit ratios are dramatically lower among people with opioid misuse or opioid use disorder (OUD) versus those without (Parker et al. 2020). Factors that may contribute to the reduced success in quitting tobacco include a higher severity of tobacco dependence and

Table 11–1. Overlap of clinical symptoms of tobacco and cannabis withdrawal

Cannabis withdrawal syndrome	Tobacco withdrawal syndrome
Irritability or aggression	**Irritability**, frustration, or anger
Nervousness or **anxiety**	**Anxiety**
Insomnia or disturbing dreams	**Insomnia**
Depressed mood	**Depressed mood**
Decreased appetite or weight loss	Increased appetite or weight gain
Restlessness	**Restlessness**
At least one physical symptom causing discomfort (i.e., abdominal pain, shakiness/tremors, sweating, fever, chills, headache)	Difficulty concentrating

high rates of chronic pain. Methadone increases cigarette consumption in a dose-dependent way (Custodio et al. 2022).

Because trials of pharmacotherapies have yielded only modest responses (Hall et al. 2018; Nahvi et al. 2014), innovative behavioral or incentive strategies will likely be needed to enhance quit smoking rates. Given the high rates of both psychiatric and personality disorders, strategies such as mindfulness, emotion regulation, and distress tolerance skills may hold promise (Cooperman et al. 2019). The opioid treatment setting can provide opportunities to access care for TUD because many people receive methadone or other medication for OUD for years, and group treatments and mutual support groups are already employed for this population. Despite the low success rates of current interventions, evidence indicates that individuals with OUD are not likely to quit smoking without treatment, thus facing almost certain early morbidity and mortality (Vlad et al. 2020).

Case Example

Lu is a 19-year-old college student who uses cigarettes, mostly on weekends. They typically smoke approximately eight cigarettes daily on Thursday, Friday, and Saturday when they go out, and none on other days of the week. They smoked intermittently in high school, and their use escalated when they started college. Sometimes they vape a pod-style electronic cigarette with friends, but they mostly use cigarettes. They almost never smoke cigarettes in the morning and almost always smoke at night, often when also drinking alcohol. They feel unable to stop and have intense cravings when out in bars or with friends, so even though they hope to stop, they find it nearly impossible. They also report vaping cannabis about twice a week, saying it helps them relax and generally feel better. Their grades were poor last year. They also report some mild anxiety but have never had any treatment for this. They feel ambivalent about stopping cannabis.

What Are the Concerns in This Case?

It is not uncommon for patients using multiple substances to have different levels of motivation about each. Lu seems most willing to work on cigarette use, which can be prioritized in terms of treatment goals. Even someone who does not smoke early in the morning or in a daily fashion can be addicted to tobacco, and, especially in younger people, the experience of not having control over cigarette use may be the determining factor in understanding the level of addiction. Goals to use NRT and to not purchase tobacco in high-risk situations, such as on the weekends, may help this patient practice abstinence. If their continued cannabis and alcohol use undermine tobacco abstinence and contribute to relapses, a plan can be discussed for temporarily reducing or avoiding these other triggers to support the primary goals. A comprehensive assessment can include mood, anxiety, and other factors that may warrant additional consideration or treatment.

Key Points

- Treatment modifications may enhance outcomes in groups with behavioral health comorbidity, but these are often modest, and usual best practices may also be appropriate.
- Illness severity and functional impairment ultimately may be more important prognostic factors than discrete diagnostic subgroups.
- Many studies have demonstrated that trying to quit smoking does not worsen mental illness, although this can be complicated in the short term by tobacco withdrawal symptoms that mimic mental illness.

- Individuals with behavioral health conditions, although motivated at similar levels to other populations, have greater difficulty quitting and less success on a given attempt, necessitating more quit attempts and perhaps longer periods of treatment.
- Modifications to counseling generally include more sessions overall, more sessions before the quit date, and a flexible quit date. Additional considerations can include more relapse prevention counseling sessions or ongoing peer support.
- Co-use of cannabis complicates tobacco cessation in ways that are not fully understood, and more studies are needed. All patients who smoke should also be screened for cannabis use.

References

Allen MH, Debanné M, Lazignac C, et al: Effect of nicotine replacement therapy on agitation in smokers with schizophrenia: a double-blind, randomized, placebo-controlled study. Am J Psychiatry 168(4):395–399, 2011 21245085

American Psychiatric Association: Diagnostic and Statistical Manual of Mental Disorders, 5th Edition, Text Revision. Washington, DC, American Psychiatric Association, 2022

Anthenelli RM, Benowitz NL, West R, et al: Neuropsychiatric safety and efficacy of varenicline, bupropion, and nicotine patch in smokers with and without psychiatric disorders (EAGLES): a double-blind, randomised, placebo-controlled clinical trial. Lancet 387(10037):2507–2520, 2016 27116918

Anthenelli RM, Gaffney M, Benowitz NL, et al: Predictors of neuropsychiatric adverse events with smoking cessation medications in the randomized controlled EAGLES trial. J Gen Intern Med 34(6):862–870, 2019 30847828

Apollonio D, Philipps R, Bero L: Interventions for tobacco use cessation in people in treatment for or recovery from substance use disorders. Cochrane Database Syst Rev 11(11):CD010274, 2016 27878808

Ayers CR, Heffner JL, Russ C, et al: Efficacy and safety of pharmacotherapies for smoking cessation in anxiety disorders: subgroup analysis of the randomized, active- and placebo-controlled EAGLES trial. Depress Anxiety 37(3):247–260, 2020 31850603

Baker AL, Borland R, Bonevski B, et al: "Quitlink": a randomized controlled trial of peer worker facilitated quitline support for smokers receiving mental health services: study protocol. Front Psychiatry 10:124, 2019 30941063

Berg SA, Sentir AM, Cooley BS, et al: Nicotine is more addictive, not more cognitively therapeutic in a neurodevelopmental model of schizophrenia produced by neonatal ventral hippocampal lesions. Addict Biol 19(6):1020–1031, 2014 23919443

Brown RA, Minami H, Hecht J, et al: Sustained care smoking cessation intervention for individuals hospitalized for psychiatric disorders: the Helping Hand 3 randomized clinical trial. JAMA Psychiatry 78(8):839–847, 2021

Brunette MF, Pratt SI, Bartels SJ, et al: Randomized trial of interventions for smoking cessation among Medicaid beneficiaries with mental illness. Psychiatr Serv 69(3):274–280, 2018 29137560

Carpenter KM, Nash CM, Vargas-Belcher RA, et al: Feasibility and early outcomes of a tailored quitline protocol for smokers with mental health conditions. Nicotine Tob Res 21(5):584–591, 2019 30768203

Chambers RA: Adult hippocampal neurogenesis in the pathogenesis of addiction and dual diagnosis disorders. Drug Alcohol Depend 130(1–3):1–12, 2013 23279925

Cooperman NA, Rizvi SL, Hughes CD, et al: Field test of a dialectical behavior therapy skills training-based intervention for smoking cessation and opioid relapse prevention in methadone treatment. J Dual Diagn 15(1):67–73, 2019 30646819

Corvin A, O'Mahony E, O'Regan M, et al: Cigarette smoking and psychotic symptoms in bipolar affective disorder. Br J Psychiatry 179:35–38, 2001 11435266

Coustals N, Martelli C, Brunet-Lecomte M, et al: Chronic smoking and cognition in patients with schizophrenia: a meta-analysis. Schizophr Res 222:113–121, 2020 32507373

Custodio L, Malone S, Bardo MT, et al: Nicotine and opioid co-dependence: findings from bench research to clinical trials. Neurosci Biobehav Rev 134:104507, 2022 34968525

de Leon J, Diaz FJ: A meta-analysis of worldwide studies demonstrates an association between schizophrenia and tobacco smoking behaviors. Schizophr Res 76(2–3):135–157, 2005 15949648

Evins AE, Benowitz NL, West R, et al: Neuropsychiatric safety and efficacy of varenicline, bupropion, and nicotine patch in smokers with psychotic, anxiety, and mood disorders in the EAGLES trial. J Clin Psychopharmacol 39(2):108–116, 2019 30811371

Evins AE, Cather C, Pratt SA, et al: Maintenance treatment with varenicline for smoking cessation in patients with schizophrenia and bipolar disorder: a randomized clinical trial. JAMA 311(2):145–154, 2014 24399553

Fischler PV, Soyka M, Seifritz E, et al: Off-label and investigational drugs in the treatment of alcohol use disorder: a critical review. Front Pharmacol 13:927703, 2022 36263121

Fitzke RE, Davis JP, Pedersen ER: Co-use of tobacco products and cannabis among veterans: a preliminary investigation of prevalence and associations with mental health outcomes. J Psychoactive Drugs 54(3):250–257, 2022 34334112

Fornaro M, Carvalho AF, De Prisco M, et al: The prevalence, odds, predictors, and management of tobacco use disorder or nicotine dependence among people with severe mental illness: systematic review and meta-analysis. Neurosci Biobehav Rev 132:289–303, 2022 34838527

Garey L, Olofsson H, Garza T, et al: The role of anxiety in smoking onset, severity, and cessation-related outcomes: a review of recent literature. Curr Psychiatry Rep 22(8):38, 2020 32506166

Gilbody S, Peckham E, Bailey D, et al: Smoking cessation for people with severe mental illness (SCIMITAR+): a pragmatic randomised controlled trial. Lancet Psychiatry 6(5):379–390, 2019 30975539

Glasheen C, Hedden SL, Forman-Hoffman VL, et al: Cigarette smoking behaviors among adults with serious mental illness in a nationally representative sample. Ann Epidemiol 24(10):776–780, 2014 25169683

Goodwin RD, Pacek LR, Copeland J, et al: Trends in daily cannabis use among cigarette smokers: United States, 2002–2014. Am J Public Health 108(1):137–142, 2018 29161058

Goodwin RD, Shevorykin A, Carl E, et al: Daily cannabis use is a barrier to tobacco cessation among tobacco quitline callers at 7-month follow-up. Nicotine Tob Res 24(10):1684–1688, 2022 35417562

Gray KM, Sonne SC, McClure EA, et al: A randomized placebo-controlled trial of N-acetylcysteine for cannabis use disorder in adults. Drug Alcohol Depend 177:249–257, 2017 28623823

Gray KM, Baker NL, McClure EA, et al: Efficacy and safety of varenicline for adolescent smoking cessation: a randomized clinical trial. JAMA Pediatr 173(12):1146–1153, 2019 31609433

Guo K, Li J, Li J, et al: The effects of pharmacological interventions on smoking cessation in people with alcohol dependence: a systematic review and meta-analysis of nine randomized controlled trials. Int J Clin Pract 75(11):e14594, 2021 34228852

Haas AL, Muñoz RF, Humfleet GL, et al: Influences of mood, depression history, and treatment modality on outcomes in smoking cessation. J Consult Clin Psychol 72(4):563–570, 2004 15301640

Hall SM, Humfleet GL, Gasper JJ, et al: Cigarette smoking cessation intervention for buprenorphine treatment patients. Nicotine Tob Res 20(5):628–635, 2018 28549161

Han ES, Foulds J, Steinberg MB, et al: Characteristics and smoking cessation outcomes of patients returning for repeat tobacco dependence treatment. Int J Clin Pract 60(9):1068–1074, 2006 16939548

Heffner JL, Strawn JR, DelBello MP, et al: The co-occurrence of cigarette smoking and bipolar disorder: phenomenology and treatment considerations. Bipolar Disord 13(5–6):439–453, 2011 22017214

Heffner JL, Evins AE, Russ C, et al: Safety and efficacy of first-line smoking cessation pharmacotherapies in bipolar disorders: subgroup analysis of a randomized clinical trial. J Affect Disord 256:267–277, 2019 31195244

Howes S, Hartmann-Boyce J, Livingstone-Banks J, et al: Antidepressants for smoking cessation. Cochrane Database Syst Rev 4(4):CD000031, 2020 32319681

Hughes JR, Stead LF, Lancaster T: Anxiolytics and antidepressants for smoking cessation. Cochrane Database Syst Rev (2):CD000031, 2000 10796472

Hughes JR, Callas PW: Past alcohol problems do not predict worse smoking cessation outcomes. Drug Alcohol Depend 71(3):269–273, 2003 12957344

Hurt RD, Offord KP, Croghan IT, et al: Mortality following inpatient addictions treatment: role of tobacco use in a community-based cohort. JAMA 275(14):1097–1103, 1996 8601929

Joseph AM, Willenbring ML, Nugent SM, et al: A randomized trial of concurrent versus delayed smoking intervention for patients in alcohol dependence treatment. J Stud Alcohol 65(6):681–691, 2004 15700504

Kessler RC, Andrews G, Colpe LJ, et al: Short screening scales to monitor population prevalences and trends in non-specific psychological distress. Psychol Med 32(6):959–976, 2002 12214795

Mallet J, Godin O, Dansou Y, et al: Current (but not ex) cigarette smoking is associated with worse cognitive performances in schizophrenia: results from the FACE-SZ cohort. Psychol Med 53(11):5279–5290, 2022 36073848

McClure EA, Tomko RL, Salazar CA, et al: Tobacco and cannabis co-use: drug substitution, quit interest, and cessation preferences. Exp Clin Psychopharmacol 27(3):265–275, 2019 30556733

McClure EA, Baker NL, Hood CO, et al: Cannabis and alcohol co-use in a smoking cessation pharmacotherapy trial for adolescents and emerging adults. Nicotine Tob Res 22(8):1374–1382, 2020 31612956

McFall M, Saxon AJ, Malte CA, et al: Integrating tobacco cessation into mental health care for posttraumatic stress disorder: a randomized controlled trial. JAMA 304(22):2485–2493, 2010 21139110

McKelvey K, Thrul J, Ramo D: Impact of quitting smoking and smoking cessation treatment on substance use outcomes: an updated and narrative review. Addict Behav 65:161–170, 2017 27816663

Mitchell JM, Teague CH, Kayser AS, et al: Varenicline decreases alcohol consumption in heavy-drinking smokers. Psychopharmacology (Berl) 223(3):299–306, 2012 22547331

Nahvi S, Ning Y, Segal KS, et al: Varenicline efficacy and safety among methadone maintained smokers: a randomized placebo-controlled trial. Addiction 109(9):1554–1563, 2014 24862167

Oon-Arom A, Likhitsathain S, Srisurapanont M: Efficacy and acceptability of varenicline for alcoholism: a systematic review and meta-analysis of randomized-controlled trials. Drug Alcohol Depend 205:107631, 2019 31678838

Pacchiarotti I, Bond DJ, Baldessarini RJ, et al: The International Society for Bipolar Disorders (ISBD) task force report on antidepressant use in bipolar disorders. Am J Psychiatry 170(11):1249–1262, 2013 24030475

Parker MA, Weinberger AH, Villanti AC: Quit ratios for cigarette smoking among individuals with opioid misuse and opioid use disorder in the United States. Drug Alcohol Depend 214:108164, 2020 32652375

Parker MA, Cordoba-Grueso WS, Streck JM, et al: Intersectionality of serious psychological distress, cigarette smoking, and substance use disorders in the United States: 2008–2018. Drug Alcohol Depend 228:109095, 2021 34601273

Piper ME, Cook JW, Schlam TR, et al: Anxiety diagnoses in smokers seeking cessation treatment: relations with tobacco dependence, withdrawal, outcome and response to treatment. Addiction 106(2):418–427, 2011 20973856

Prochaska JJ, Delucchi K, Hall SM: A meta-analysis of smoking cessation interventions with individuals in substance abuse treatment or recovery. J Consult Clin Psychol 72(6):1144–1156, 2004a 15612860

Prochaska JJ, Gill P, Hall SM: Treatment of tobacco use in an inpatient psychiatric setting. Psychiatr Serv 55(11):1265–1270, 2004b 15534015

Quisenberry AJ, Pittman J, Goodwin RD, et al: Smoking relapse risk is increased among individuals in recovery. Drug Alcohol Depend 202:93–103, 2019 31325822

Richter KP, McCool RM, Okuyemi KS, et al: Patients' views on smoking cessation and tobacco harm reduction during drug treatment. Nicotine Tob Res 4(Suppl 2):S175–S182, 2002 12573178

Rosen RL, Ramasubramani RS, Benowitz NL, et al: Caffeine levels and dietary intake in smokers with schizophrenia and bipolar disorder. Psychiatry Res 319:114989, 2023 36470161

Siru R, Hulse GK, Tait RJ: Assessing motivation to quit smoking in people with mental illness: a review. Addiction 104(5):719–733, 2009 19413788

Taylor G, McNeill A, Girling A, et al: Change in mental health after smoking cessation: systematic review and meta-analysis. BMJ 348:g1151, 2014 24524926

Taylor GM, Lindson N, Farley A, et al: Smoking cessation for improving mental health. Cochrane Database Syst Rev 3(3):CD013522, 2021 33687070

Thurgood SL, McNeill A, Clark-Carter D, et al: A systematic review of smoking cessation interventions for adults in substance abuse treatment or recovery. Nicotine Tob Res 18(5):993–1001, 2016 26069036

Tidey JW, Colby SM, Xavier EM: Effects of smoking abstinence on cigarette craving, nicotine withdrawal, and nicotine reinforcement in smokers with and without schizophrenia. Nicotine Tob Res 16(3):326–334, 2014 24113929

Tsoi DT, Porwal M, Webster AC: Interventions for smoking cessation and reduction in individuals with schizophrenia. Cochrane Database Syst Rev 2013(2):CD007253, 2013 23450574

Vanable PA, Carey MP, Carey KB, et al: Smoking among psychiatric outpatients: relationship to substance use, diagnosis, and illness severity. Psychol Addict Behav 17(4):259–265, 2003 14640821

van Amsterdam J, van den Brink W: The effect of alcohol use on smoking cessation: a systematic review. Alcohol 109:13–22, 2023

van der Meer RM, Willemsen MC, Smit F, et al: Smoking cessation interventions for smokers with current or past depression. Cochrane Database Syst Rev 8(8):CD006102, 2013 23963776

Vlad C, Arnsten JH, Nahvi S: Achieving smoking cessation among persons with opioid use disorder. CNS Drugs 34(4):367–387, 2020 32107731

Weinberger AH, Desai RA, McKee SA: Nicotine withdrawal in U.S. smokers with current mood, anxiety, alcohol use, and substance use disorders. Drug Alcohol Depend 108(1–2):7–12, 2010 20006451

Weinberger AH, Gbedemah M, Goodwin RD: Cigarette smoking quit rates among adults with and without alcohol use disorders and heavy alcohol use, 2002–2015: a representative sample of the United States population. Drug Alcohol Depend 180:204–207, 2017a 28918239

Weinberger AH, Kashan RS, Shpigel DM, et al: Depression and cigarette smoking behavior: a critical review of population-based studies. Am J Drug Alcohol Abuse 43(4):416–431, 2017b 27286288

Weinberger AH, Pacek LR, Giovenco D, et al: Cigarette use among individuals with alcohol use disorders in the United States, 2002 to 2016: trends overall and by race/ethnicity. Alcohol (Hanover) 43(1):79–90, 2019 30408209

Weinberger AH, Pacek LR, Wall MM, et al: Cigarette smoking quit ratios among adults in the USA with cannabis use and cannabis use disorders, 2002–2016. Tob Control 29(1):74–80, 2020 30952691

Weinberger AH, Zhu J, Lee J, et al: Cannabis use and the onset of cigarette and e-cigarette use: a prospective, longitudinal study among youth in the United States. Nicotine Tob Res 23(3):609–613, 2021 32835370

West R, Evins AE, Benowitz NL, et al: Factors associated with the efficacy of smoking cessation treatments and predictors of smoking abstinence in EAGLES. Addiction 113(8):1507–1516, 2018 29508470

Williams JM, Foulds J: Successful tobacco dependence treatment in schizophrenia. Am J Psychiatry 164(2):222–227, quiz 373, 2007 17267783

Williams JM, Ziedonis DM, Vreeland B, et al: A wellness approach to addressing tobacco in mental health settings: Learning About Healthy Living. Am J Psychiatr Rehabil 12(4):352–369, 2009

Williams JM, Steinberg ML, Zimmermann MH, et al: Comparison of two intensities of tobacco dependence counseling in schizophrenia and schizoaffective disorder. J Subst Abuse Treat 38(4):384–393, 2010 20363089

Williams JM, Gandhi KK, Lu S-E, et al: Shorter interpuff interval is associated with higher nicotine intake in smokers with schizophrenia. Drug Alcohol Depend 118(2–3):313–319, 2011 21596491

Williams JM, Anthenelli RM, Morris CD, et al: A randomized, double-blind, placebo-controlled study evaluating the safety and efficacy of varenicline for smoking cessation in patients with schizophrenia or schizoaffective disorder. J Clin Psychiatry 73(5):654–660, 2012 22697191

Winhusen TM, Brigham GS, Kropp F, et al: A randomized trial of concurrent smoking-cessation and substance use disorder treatment in stimulant-dependent smokers. J Clin Psychiatry 75(4):336–343, 2014 24345356

12

Switching From Smoked to Non-Smoked Nicotine Products

As outlined in Chapter 1, most of our knowledge about the harms to health from tobacco and about treatment for tobacco use disorder (TUD) is based on studies of people who smoke cigarettes. However, as summarized in Chapter 2, by 2020 electronic (e-)cigarettes had become the second most commonly used tobacco product among adults after cigarettes (12.5% vs. 3.7%) (Cornelius et al. 2022), and cigars, e-cigarettes, and smokeless tobacco were all being used by more than 4% of male tobacco users. However, product use among teenagers and young adults is often predictive of future patterns, and in both of these groups, e-cigarettes are now more commonly used than cigarettes. For example, among 18- to 24-year-olds in 2020, 7.4% were using cigarettes, 9.4% were using e-cigarettes, and 5.7% were using two or more products (Cornelius et al. 2022).

FDA Regulation and Its Effects

Regulatory developments by the FDA Center for Tobacco Products (FDA-CTP) are indicative of the FDA's view of the relative harmfulness of different products and may have an important impact on future patterns of nontherapeutic nicotine product use. In 2009, the Tobacco Control Act gave manufacturers the opportunity to apply for their product to be authorized as a "modified-risk tobacco product" (MRTP). These applications must contain comprehensive data supporting potential claims that the product is either less harmful to health than regular cigarettes or that, when normally used, it delivers a lower level of toxicants than is typically delivered by cigarettes. This application requires a higher burden of proof than is currently required for a "premarket tobacco product application" (PMTA), which requires a company to demonstrate that marketing of any new product not on the market in 2007 is "appropriate for the protection of public health." Products given marketing authorization by the FDA may then apply for an MRTP (Solyst 2023). From 2011 to 2022, 47 MRTP applications were filed with the FDA, and 15 "modified risk granted orders" (MRGOs) were authorized. However, to date, these MRTP authorizations really apply only to different subtypes of the following three products:

- General Snus, a form of oral tobacco manufactured by Swedish Match (now owned by Philip Morris International), was given an MRGO in 2019. This allowed the manufacturers to include the following risk information in their product marketing: "Using General Snus instead of cigarettes puts you at a lower risk of mouth cancer, heart disease, lung cancer, stroke, emphysema, and chronic bronchitis."
- IQOS, a brand of "heat-not-burn" cigarette manufactured by Phillip Morris International, was granted an MRGO in 2020, and modified versions were authorized in 2021 and 2023. This authorized IQOS marketing to state: "The IQOS system heats tobacco but does not burn it. This significantly reduces the production of harmful and potentially harmful chemicals. Scientific studies have shown that switching completely from conventional cigarettes to the IQOS system significantly reduces your body's exposure to harmful or potentially harmful chemicals."

- VLN King, a brand of very low nicotine content cigarettes manufactured by 22nd Century Group that contain approximately 95% less nicotine than most cigarette brands, was granted an MRGO in 2020. This authorized the marketing for VLN King products to state: 1) "95% less nicotine"; 2) "helps reduce your nicotine consumption"; and 3) "greatly reduces your nicotine consumption."

Thousands of traditional cigarette and cigar products that were on the market before 2007 were allowed to remain on the market simply by providing evidence about their constituents and by demonstrating that the products currently on the market are "substantially equivalent" to those on the market prior to 2007 (Carpenter et al. 2017). Thousands of these highly dangerous products were "grandfathered in" in this way, despite clear evidence that they increase fatalities among long-term regular users and cause numerous serious diseases.

Regulation of Electronic Cigarettes

E-cigarettes are electronic devices that transform a liquid containing nicotine into an aerosol that is inhaled via a mouthpiece (Pesko et al. 2023). Because e-cigarettes were not being widely marketed when the 2009 Tobacco Control Act was signed into law, these and other newer products were later (2016) formally deemed as being "tobacco products" under the Act and had until 2020 to submit a PMTA to remain on the market (pending the FDA's decision on each application). More than 6.6 million individual e-cigarette product applications were submitted (including individual liquid flavors, devices, and chargers), and as of early 2023, more than 99% of these had been denied. Some of the brands with the largest market share are still being assessed, but to date, only seven e-cigarette devices, made by three companies, have received marketing orders. Although many (likely millions) of PMTA applications were for different e-liquids containing different nicotine concentrations, additives, and flavors, at this time the only e-liquid flavors that have been authorized are those with "tobacco" or menthol flavor. It appears likely that the FDA considers e-cigarette liquids with flavors other than tobacco to be attractive to people younger than 21, so any potential public health benefits of adults switching to that brand of e-cigarette may be offset by the potential public health harms resulting from young people initiating the use of such products because they are attracted by the flavor.

Proposed Future FDA Regulatory Actions

Since the 2009 Tobacco Control Act, it has been very difficult to predict future FDA regulatory actions on tobacco, and even harder to predict the actual implementation dates of regulatory actions that have been publicly announced by the FDA-CTP. For example, when the 2009 Act was passed into law, two regulatory actions near the top of the agenda were 1) implementing pictorial warning labels on cigarette packs (Kaufman et al. 2022) and 2) banning menthol as a characterizing flavor in cigarettes (Stephenson 2022). Largely as a result of legal opposition by the tobacco companies, as of 2024 (more than 15 years later), neither of these policies has been implemented.

Despite this continuing difficulty in predicting which proposed FDA regulatory actions actually will be implemented in the near future, two major regulatory actions have been proposed repeatedly and appear likely to be implemented at some point within the next 10 years:

1. **Ban menthol as a characterizing flavor in cigarettes** (and all characterizing flavors (other than tobacco) in cigars (Stephenson 2022).

If implemented, the menthol ban will force current menthol cigarette users to make one of the following choices: 1) switch to non-mentholated cigarettes; 2) quit tobacco completely; 3) quit smoking menthols by switching to a much less harmful, non-smoked nicotine product; or 4) attempt to continue smoking menthol flavor by purchasing smuggled/illicit menthol tobacco products. Of these options, quitting tobacco completely is clearly the best for health. Neither switching to non-mentholated cigarettes nor using illicit products has any health benefit. Switching to a less harmful, non-smoked product offers the best option for those who continue to use nicotine and poses a significantly reduced harm to health. When the ban on menthol as a characterizing flavor in smoked tobacco is implemented, there likely will be an increase in people seeking to quit smoking or to change their smoking behavior. This will particularly affect Black/ African American people who smoke (of whom more than 80% smoke menthol brands; Lawrence et al. 2010), and menthol-flavored cigarettes are also more popular among young people and females. It is important that when the menthol ban is implemented, health professionals will be ready to assist the users of these products in making healthier choices, even if that involves continuing to use non-smoked products.

2. **Require permissible nicotine content in cigarettes and other combusted products to be reduced to nonaddictive levels** (approximately 95% reduction in nicotine content).

This proposal has been supported by two consecutive U.S. administrations (Trump and Biden) (Gottlieb and Zeller 2017), and its perceived feasibility may change if New Zealand implements a similar regulation (Foulds et al. 2022b), which has been passed into law in that country and was proposed to be implemented fully by 2025. The reduced nicotine strategy is clearly much more ambitious than other potential FDA product standards because it will likely have a major impact on sales of the most widely used tobacco product: cigarettes. When implemented, this regulation will again give users options:

- Switch to legal, very low nicotine content cigarettes;
- Quit tobacco completely;
- Quit smoking combusted tobacco products by switching to a much less harmful (non-smoked) nicotine product; or
- Attempt to continue smoking high nicotine cigarettes/cigars by purchasing smuggled/illicit high nicotine smoked tobacco products.

Of these options, again, quitting tobacco completely is clearly the best for health, followed by switching to a less harmful (non-smoked) product. Neither switching to very low nicotine cigarettes nor using illicit products will benefit users' health, and the former will likely prove very difficult for people addicted to smoking because they will find that their very low nicotine cigarettes are less satisfying and reinforcing, which will likely result in lower cigarette consumption even if the person is not planning to reduce or quit.

A large number of randomized trials of very low nicotine cigarettes have been completed, and these generally found that when people switched to very low nicotine cigarettes, they reduced their smoke intake (rather than increasing smoking). Although they do experience some nicotine withdrawal symptoms during the first few weeks, they become less addicted to cigarettes over time (Donny and White 2022). One particular trial in people with mood or anxiety disorders found no evidence of worsening mental health while switching to very low nicotine cigarettes and reported that more participants successfully quit smoking when offered brief counseling and nicotine replacement therapy (NRT) (Foulds et al. 2022b).

Implementation of the reduced nicotine standard likely will produce a significant reduction in cigarette smoking and an enormous long-term improvement in public health (Apelberg et al. 2018). It also will likely result in a large increase in demand for smoking cessation assistance, and because some people will likely switch to another nicotine product long-term, health professionals will need to be able to provide accurate advice on the relative harms to health from these alternative products.

Switching to Less Harmful Tobacco Products

There is a broad consensus within the public health community that combustible tobacco products (e.g., cigarettes and cigars) are more harmful to health than non-combusted nicotine products (e.g., snus, e-cigarettes, heat-not-burn products) (Centers for Disease Control and Prevention, National Center for Chronic Disease Prevention and Health Promotion, Office on Smoking and Health 2010). If some people who smoke, particularly those who are not currently planning to quit or do not want to use current evidence-based treatments (e.g., varenicline, bupropion, NRT), could successfully switch to a significantly less harmful nicotine product, that would likely result in reduced harm for both that individual and for society.

Smokeless Tobacco/Snus for Smoking Cessation

Considerable evidence suggests that the form of smokeless tobacco called snus has helped many Swedish males to switch completely from smoked tobacco and ultimately to quit smoking (Foulds et al. 2003; Ramström and Foulds 2006). A systematic review and meta-analysis published in 2022 concluded that,

> While the meta-analysis of [randomized controlled trials] did not show
> a significant association between snus use and smoking cessation, the
> results of the meta-analysis of longitudinal cohort studies (RR 1.38,
> 95% CI 1.05–1.82, *P*=0.022) and cross-sectional studies (OR 1.87, 95% CI
> 1.29–2.72, *P*=0.001) indicated that use of snus was associated with an
> increased likelihood of quitting or having quit smoking. (Stjepanović
> et al. 2023, p. 757)

Therefore, the evidence from randomized controlled trials showing
that snus helps people quit smoking remains weak, so in clinical practice, patients first should be offered approved medicines. However,
patients who are very reluctant to use a medicine for smoking cessation
and who are interested in trying a smokeless tobacco product could
reasonably try one of the General Snus products that have been given
an MRTP designation by the FDA. It should be noted that such a designation does not signify FDA approval as a cessation aid but at least
indicates that, after reviewing considerable data, the FDA considers the
product to be less harmful than cigarettes.

Electronic Cigarettes for Smoking Cessation

The Cochrane Review of e-cigarettes for smoking cessation (as of early
2024; this is a living review), concluded that

> There is high-certainty evidence that electronic cigarettes (ECs) with
> nicotine increase quit rates compared to NRT and moderate-certainty
> evidence that they increase quit rates compared to ECs without nico-
> tine. Evidence comparing nicotine EC with usual care/no treatment
> also suggests benefit. (Lindson et al. 2024)

The data included in that review included both a randomized, placebo-controlled trial of e-cigarettes in participants not planning to quit
smoking (Foulds et al. 2022a) and a longitudinal cohort study of people
also not planning to quit (Kasza et al. 2021). In the trial by Foulds et
al. (2022a), participants were randomly assigned to using 1) a plastic
tube with the appearance and feel of a cigarette to replace behavioral
characteristics; 2) a zero-nicotine e-cigarette; 3) an 8-mg/mL nicotine
e-cigarette; or 4) a 36-mg/mL nicotine e-cigarette. Participants were
encouraged to reduce their smoking by 50% and then by 75% over the
first month and to replace some cigarettes with use of their assigned

products. The proportion in each group who had quit smoking during the 6 months is shown in Figure 12–1.

Although the quit rate in the high-nicotine e-cigarette group at 6 months was not high (11%), it was significantly higher than in the cigarette substitute (3%) or the placebo e-cigarette (1%) groups. The

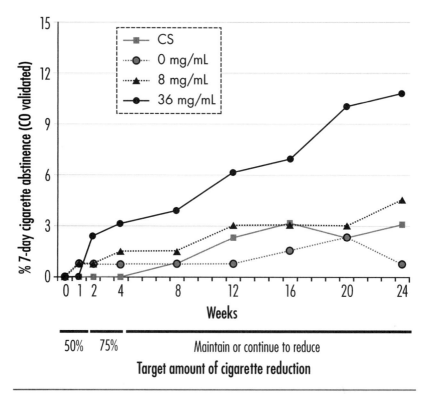

Figure 12–1. Percentage of participants in each randomly assigned group reporting zero cigarette consumption in the prior 7 days at eight follow-up visits, validated by exhaled carbon monoxide <10 ppm, at each visit (0-mg/mL, 8-mg/mL, or 36-mg/mL nicotine concentration in an electronic nicotine delivery system or cigarette substitute [CS]).

CO = carbon monoxide.

Source. Foulds J, Cobb CO, Yen M-S, et al: "Effect of Electronic Nicotine Delivery Systems on Cigarette Abstinence in Smokers With No Plans to Quit: Exploratory Analysis of a Randomized Placebo-Controlled Trial." *Nicotine and Tobacco Research* 24(7):955–961, 2022. This article is licensed under a Creative Commons Attribution 4.0 International License (https://creativecommons.org /licenses/by/4.0).

fact that the 8-mg/mL nicotine e-cigarette did not result in many participants quitting shows that having nicotine delivery close to that of a cigarette may be important for e-cigarettes to help people trying to quit. It should be acknowledged that in trials like this one, the products are given for free and the participants are encouraged to reduce smoking throughout the trial (but not quit), aspects that are very different from the world outside of clinical trials. However, the studies by Kasza et al. (2021, 2023) and other studies of people using e-cigarettes have also found that those not planning to quit are more likely to achieve smoking abstinence a year later if they use a nicotine e-cigarette on a daily basis.

No e-cigarette products have received an MRTP designation from the FDA-CTP as of August 2024, and none has applied for approval from the FDA Center for Drug Evaluation and Research as a smoking cessation drug or device. Given that relatively few e-cigarette products have received marketing authorization from the FDA, MRTP authorization does not seem to be on the horizon, and it is unlikely that approval as a cessation product will even be applied for in the near future. Nonetheless, there is high public interest in using these products in place of cigarettes in many countries, and the evidence suggests that such products can help people quit smoking without causing serious adverse events. There is also evidence that switching from smoking to vaping or dual use appears to significantly reduce levels of biomarkers of potential harm (Hartmann-Boyce et al. 2023).

Given that a very small proportion of products that were launched on the market have received FDA marketing authorization, it would seem preferable, if asked, to recommend that a patient who smokes try an e-cigarette product that has FDA marketing authorization because this means that the manufacturer has attempted to conduct itself within the legal framework provided by the FDA; has provided a considerable amount of data on the quality of the product, its toxicant emissions, and so on, to the FDA; and is less likely than non-authorized products to be removed from the market by the FDA. The choices at present are limited to a handful of products, and not all have published details on their basic characteristics (e.g., nicotine pharmacokinetics). However, one published example that is fairly typical of current e-cigarettes is the Vuse Solo, which has been studied with 57-mg/mL nicotine salt liquid in a cartridge. Figure 12–2 shows the blood nicotine levels produced by 10 minutes of *ad libitum* puffing compared with the same puffing on participants' usual brand of cigarette or 30 minutes chewing 4-mg nicotine gum (GSK brand) (Campbell et al. 2022). As is typical of

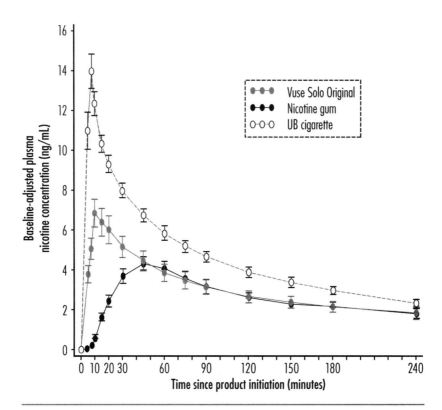

Figure 12–2. Mean baseline-adjusted plasma nicotine concentration profiles from use of (a) Vuse Solo "Original" electronic cigarette with liquid nicotine concentration 57 mg/mL, (b) 4-mg nicotine gum, or (c) usual brand (UB) traditional cigarette.

Source.   Campbell C, Jin T, Round EK, et al: "Part One: Abuse Liability of Vuse Solo (G2) Electronic Nicotine Delivery System Relative to Combustible Cigarettes and Nicotine Gum." *Scientific Reports* 12(1):22080, 2022. This article is licensed under a Creative Commons Attribution 4.0 International License (https://creativecommons.org/licenses/by/4.0).

most e-cigarettes, the nicotine delivery is faster and higher than from nicotine replacement, but lower than from smoking a cigarette. This, together with the behavioral and sensory similarities to smoking, is likely why e-cigarettes have greater appeal and possibly efficacy for smoking cessation than NRT.

As of 2024, there is no conclusive evidence regarding the use of other non-smoked tobacco products as a tool to help people quit smoking cigarettes. For example, although new products such as heat-not-burn cigarettes or nicotine pouches (containing no tobacco) may appear to have similar characteristics to e-cigarettes or smokeless tobacco, there is insufficient evidence to guide their use in clinical practice.

Perhaps the main challenge when considering recommending the use of any of these products is that, because they do not have authorization for a smoking cessation indication, they provide no or minimal advice on the label for that purpose. Patients are left to figure out the dosing for themselves via trial and error or by searching on the internet for clues and advice from experienced users. Another challenge is that, with the exception of snus/smokeless tobacco, which has fairly thorough long-term epidemiology, there is a lack of knowledge regarding the long-term health effects of these products. For these reasons, it is understandable that most clinicians continue to recommend approved smoking cessation products as first- and second-line treatments and to only consider non-smoked tobacco products for patients who show a particular interest and have not succeeded in quitting with approved medicines.

Helping Patients to Quit Non-Cigarette Products

As described in Chapter 2, the trend in most high-income countries (e.g., Canada, United Kingdom, United States) is for cigarette smoking rates to be in decline and for the use of other tobacco/nicotine products to be gradually increasing. This implies that in future years clinicians may be asked more frequently to help patients quit their e-cigarettes, heat-not-burn products, or smokeless tobacco products. (There is a longer experience with helping smokeless tobacco users to quit.) As with cigarettes, there is evidence that behavioral interventions can be effective (Nethan et al. 2020) and that varenicline and NRT work in a manner similar to their role in smoking cessation (Ebbert et al. 2015).

A few trials of e-cigarette cessation interventions have been conducted, with promising results, for a cell phone texting-based intervention for young e-cigarette users (Graham et al. 2021) and pilot interventions using adapted telephone quitline protocols for tobacco cessation among people who smoke and use e-cigarettes (Carpenter et al. 2019). Until we have more definitive evidence, clinicians should assess dependence on any nicotine products as described in Chapter 4 and assess motivation to quit as described in Chapter 6. The main additional issue in the case of someone attempting to quit a non-smoked product is assessment of their likelihood or risk of relapsing back to smoking. For people who have never smoked or who quit smoking years ago, this risk may be very small, but for people who have a long history of cigarette smoking and have only completely switched to another nicotine product in the past year or two, relapsing back to smoking is a real concern. Given that relapsing could result in a substantial worsening of health risks and outcomes, such patients should be informed that the most important thing for their health is that they stay off cigarettes and that there is likely no rush to quit non-smoked products until they feel ready to do so. If the patient has their own personal reason for wanting to quit all nicotine products as soon as possible (e.g., planning to start a family, aware of increased cardiovascular problems), then an adaptation of treatment that is effective for cigarettes (e.g., counseling plus medication) is a reasonable place to start. Telephone quitline services in most countries have considerable experience with helping callers to quit numerous nicotine products and are already developing product-specific protocols, so although these services are often considered "smokers' quitlines," they typically will help callers who use any nicotine product.

Case Example

Mary (age 28) started smoking at age 15, increasing to 20 cigarettes a day (a pack) in college and continuing to smoke after college despite numerous quit attempts, partly due to the stress of her successful marketing career. She finally found time for a long-term relationship and now hopes to get married and have a family. She is highly motivated to quit smoking because her partner does not smoke, and she knows the smoking would be harmful to the baby if she became pregnant. She has previously tried nicotine replacement but has never been able to quit for more than 6 weeks because she believes that cigarettes are more effective in keeping her calm and helping her focus when she has to work long hours. She has also tried varenicline but found the side effects (nausea and insomnia) too unpleasant. She is seeking advice on the use of e-cigarettes as a less harmful replacement for cigarettes.

What Are the Concerns in This Case?

The evidence suggests that most e-cigarettes deliver much lower levels of and fewer toxicants than cigarette smoking and can increase a person's chances of quitting cigarettes. However, only a few brands and liquids have been authorized by the FDA as being appropriate for the protection of public health, and even these do not have much data on the health effects of long-term use (e.g., beyond a few years). The products themselves do not come with clear guidance on "switching" or publicly available information on nicotine delivery. They also do not come with instructions for quitting the use of the e-cigarette after successfully switching from cigarettes. If Mary wants to minimize potential harms, she should quit all nicotine products prior to becoming pregnant. Once these issues have been discussed (and retreatment with approved cessation medications reconsidered), if Mary still prefers to try to quit smoking by switching to an e-cigarette, then she should be supported in this because it would likely have beneficial health effects compared with continued smoking. She should be encouraged to use an FDA-authorized product and (in the absence of other instructions) advised to use it much like nicotine replacement. She could choose between switching abruptly (as is typical with NRT) or more gradually replacing cigarettes with e-cigarette use over a few weeks. As with NRT, her chances of quitting smoking completely are better if she initially uses the e-cigarette frequently (e.g., in place of at least 50% of her cigarettes during the first week) and if she can persist in daily e-cigarette use for at least a month. She also should be offered support to withdraw from e-cigarette use whenever she is ready to do so.

Key Points

- The tobacco and nicotine marketplace is currently shifting away from smoked products and is shifting toward the use of non-smoked nicotine products.
- This shift is occurring at all ages but is particularly strong among younger age groups (e.g., younger than 25), for whom electronic cigarettes are now the most widely used nicotine product.
- The evidence is clear that non-smoked products deliver far lower numbers and concentrations of toxicants and thus are likely to be much less harmful to health than smoked products.
- Non-smoked products (e.g., electronic cigarettes, snus, nicotine pouches, heat-not-burn cigarettes) all deliver nicotine and can be addictive.
- Approved smoking cessation medications remain the first-choice forms of pharmacotherapy, but if a patient has their own reasons for switching to a non-smoked nicotine product that is

not approved for smoking cessation, this can be supported as a potential step toward harm reduction.

- Nicotine is addictive and not harmless to health, particularly in certain circumstances (e.g., pregnancy). Users of non-smoked nicotine products should be assisted in quitting those products as well when they are ready to do so.

References

Apelberg BJ, Feirman SP, Salazar E, et al: Potential public health effects of reducing nicotine levels in cigarettes in the United States. N Engl J Med 378(18):1725–1733, 2018 29543114

Campbell C, Jin T, Round EK, et al: Part one: abuse liability of Vuse Solo (G2) electronic nicotine delivery system relative to combustible cigarettes and nicotine gum. Sci Rep 12(1):22080, 2022 36543869

Carpenter D, Connolly GN, Lempert LK: Substantial equivalence standards in tobacco governance: statutory clarity and regulatory precedent for the FSPTCA. J Health Polit Policy Law 42(4):607–644, 2017 27864349

Carpenter KM, Nash CM, Vargas-Belcher RA, et al: Feasibility and early outcomes of a tailored quitline protocol for smokers with mental health conditions. Nicotine Tob Res 21(5):584–591, 2019 30768203

Centers for Disease Control and Prevention, National Center for Chronic Disease Prevention and Health Promotion, Office on Smoking and Health: How Tobacco Smoke Causes Disease: The Biology and Behavioral Basis for Smoking-Attributable Disease. A Report of the Surgeon General. Atlanta, GA, Centers for Disease Control and Prevention, 2010

Cornelius ME, Loretan CG, Wang TW, et al: Tobacco product use among adults—United States, 2020. MMWR Morb Mortal Wkly Rep 71(11):397–405, 2022 35298455

Donny EC, White CM: A review of the evidence on cigarettes with reduced addictiveness potential. Int J Drug Policy 99:103436, 2022 34535366

Ebbert JO, Elrashidi MY, Stead LF: Interventions for smokeless tobacco use cessation. Cochrane Database Syst Rev 2015(10):CD004306, 2015 26501380

Foulds J, Ramstrom L, Burke M, et al: Effect of smokeless tobacco (snus) on smoking and public health in Sweden. Tob Control 12(4):349–359, 2003 14660766

Foulds J, Cobb CO, Yen M-S, et al: Effect of electronic nicotine delivery systems on cigarette abstinence in smokers with no plans to quit: exploratory analysis of a randomized placebo-controlled trial. Nicotine Tob Res 24(7):955–961, 2022a 34850164

Foulds J, Veldheer S, Pachas G, et al: The effects of reduced nicotine content cigarettes on biomarkers of nicotine and toxicant exposure, smoking behavior and psychiatric symptoms in smokers with mood or anxiety disorders: a double-blind randomized trial. PLoS One 17(11):e0275522, 2022b 36322562

Gottlieb S, Zeller M: A nicotine-focused framework for public health. N Engl J Med 377(12):1111–1114, 2017 28813211

Graham AL, Amato MS, Cha S, et al: Effectiveness of a vaping cessation text message program among young adult e-cigarette users: a randomized clinical trial. JAMA Intern Med 181(7):923–930, 2021 33999133

Hartmann-Boyce J, Butler AR, Theodoulou A, et al: Biomarkers of potential harm in people switching from smoking tobacco to exclusive e-cigarette use, dual use or abstinence: secondary analysis of Cochrane systematic review of trials of e-cigarettes for smoking cessation. Addiction 118(3):539–545, 2023 36208090

Kasza KA, Edwards KC, Kimmel HL, et al: Association of e-cigarette use with discontinuation of cigarette smoking among adult smokers who were initially never planning to quit. JAMA Netw Open 4(12):e2140880, 2021 34962556

Kasza KA, Hammond D, Gravely S, et al: Associations between nicotine vaping uptake and cigarette smoking cessation vary by smokers' plans to quit: longitudinal findings from the International Tobacco Control Four Country Smoking and Vaping Surveys. Addiction 118(2):340–352, 2023 36110040

Kaufman AR, D'Angelo H, Gaysynsky A, et al: Public support for cigarette pack pictorial health warnings among US adults: a cross-sectional analysis of the 2020 Health Information National Trends Survey. Nicotine Tob Res 24(6):924–928, 2022 35060607

Lawrence D, Rose A, Fagan P, et al: National patterns and correlates of mentholated cigarette use in the United States. Addiction 105(Suppl 1):13–31, 2010 21059133

Lindson N, Butler AR, McRobbie H, et al: Electronic cigarettes for smoking cessation. Cochrane Database Syst Rev 1(1):CD010216, 2024 38189560

Nethan ST, Sinha DN, Sharma S, et al: Behavioral interventions for smokeless tobacco cessation. Nicotine Tob Res 22(4):588–593, 2020 31251347

Pesko MF, Cummings KM, Douglas CE, et al: United States public health officials need to correct e-cigarette health misinformation. Addiction 118(5):785–788, 2023 36507802

Ramström LM, Foulds J: Role of snus in initiation and cessation of tobacco smoking in Sweden. Tob Control 15(3):210–214, 2006 16728752

Solyst J: The importance of harmful and potentially harmful constituents in the implementation of the 2009 US Family Smoking Prevention and Tobacco Control Act. Drug Test Anal 15(10):1198–1204, 2023 36094139

Stephenson J: FDA outlines proposed ban on menthol cigarettes, flavored
    cigars. JAMA Health Forum 3(5):e221664, 2022 36219027
Stjepanović D, Phartiyal P, Leung J, et al: Efficacy of smokeless tobacco for
    smoking cessation: a systematic review and meta-analysis. Tob Control
    32(6):757–768, 2023 35197366

Index